Slimmer

'When my friend, Dr Chris [...]
Walduck when I was on a [...]
totally amazed and astonished by his accomplishments.
I've spent my whole life motivating Marines and the
general public to come out their comfort zones to achieve
maximum potential. The mission that Charlie has
accomplished is just incredible and outstanding! What a
way to really dig deep and find some intestinal fortitude.
He is a **dieting hero** in my mind and, trust me, that's not
easy! Ooh rah Charlie!'
Harvey E. Walden, *expert fitness instructor*

'Charlie's story is truly inspirational. As a professional
athlete, I know the dedication it takes to keep in peak
condition. To see someone go from not being able to walk
to shedding thirty stone and then run marathons is
testament to his determination.
Ian 'The Machine' Freeman, *professional cage fighter*

'Charlie is an inspiration and I was delighted to witness
his astonishing transformation. It is wonderful that he is
sharing his knowledge and wisdom so that he can help
transform people's lives.'
Lorraine Kelly, *TV presenter*

'Congratulations on all you have achieved.'
Tony Blair, *ex-Prime Minister*

Slimmer Charlie

Charles Walduck

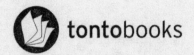

www.tontobooks.co.uk

Published in 2009 by Tonto Books Limited
Copyright © Charles Walduck 2009
All rights reserved
The moral rights of the author have been asserted

ISBN-13:
9780955632686

British Library Cataloguing-in-Publication Data:
A catalogue record for this book is available from
the British Library

Cover design & photo section by Elliot at
www.preamptive.com

Printed & bound in Great Britain
by CPI Mackays, Chatham

Tonto Books Ltd
Blaydon-on-Tyne
United Kingdom

www.tontobooks.co.uk

To Mum and Dad and my family for their unfailing
support through the dark and difficult times.

Foreword

C harlie Walduck is unlike any man I've ever known, not just for who he was, but for who he is now. Until I met him, his life had been ordinary, except for the vast amounts of food he ate every day, and his obesity problem – he weighed forty-four stone! He weighed more in stones than his age in years and was well on his way to a premature death.

He ended up as one of the UK's fattest men and had got to the point where he didn't actually think it was worth trying to lose weight and reclaim his life, body and mind. He'd resigned himself to the fact that he was too fat to bother and was beyond hope. He was addicted to food.

His closest friend sent a letter to me at ITV's *This Morning* show, where I am resident GP, and I agreed to help Charlie lose weight. We documented his progress on the show as he subsequently turned his life around. The rest of the story, as they say, is history.

Charlie lost twenty stones in the first twelve months, without the help of drugs or surgery – a UK record. He went on to lose a total of thirty-one stones, is now an inspiration to everyone who wants to lose weight. This book describes his remarkable journey and the weight loss plan that was the secret to his incredible success.

He's one of life's true heroes and certainly not the overweight loner he once thought he was. I don't know of many people in the world who could turn their entire life around for good. It amazes me that someone with such low self-esteem, no willpower, no self-confidence and clinical depression could battle his way through it all, lose a huge amount of weight and emerge as a national treasure, having touched the hearts and inspired millions of *This Morning*'s viewers as well.

I'm so proud that he followed the weight loss programme to become a new, confident Charlie, who is now himself an expert on weight loss. In this book he tells the reader how he did it. It was never going to be easy to lose such excess weight but, if Charlie did it, anyone who reads his story can lose any amount.

Charlie lost thirty-one stones and I gained a good friend ... Charlie Walduck!

Dr Chris Steele, MBE.

Preface

There we were in the hideout of the baddies. They had the girl in a separate room and I knew I was running out of time. The clock was ticking, the sweat trickling down my brow as I prepared myself for their next onslaught. The really sadistic one came at me with his fist clenched and I knew I couldn't take much punishment. I pulled on the ropes as hard as I could and my hands broke free. I was up from the chair before he knew what was going on, kicked him in the groin and floored him with a knockout punch. The two guards on the door came forward and I grabbed them and cracked their heads together. They sunk to the floor unconscious. I snatched one of their guns, kicked the door open and went looking for the girl. I knew there were less than ten seconds to find her and deactivate the missile ...

You always remember the big highs and lows in your life; where you were when something important happened in the world and who you were with. In my thirty-five years there weren't that many highs to recall, just the lows that seemed to be there constantly.

New Year's Eve 2002 is one of those times I remember with great sadness. Rather than being with people and celebrating, I was alone in my house as usual; a single man, hardly able to walk, struggling to get out of bed, go to the toilet and weighing an incredible forty-five stones, maybe more. I'd stopped paying attention to the numbers. They didn't mean anything anymore.

My constant companion on this night was the old faithful – my fridge – which was crammed full of unhealthy fattening food; all the kinds of things you are told not to eat, comfort eating at its very finest. And there was a carrier bag more of it, stuffed full of sweets, crisps, cakes, bread and cheese, next to my chair so I'd just have to reach down for my next fix. Discarded wrappers from all the rubbish I'd devoured throughout the day lay strewn across the floor in typical 'pig-sty' fashion. I'm not a messy person by nature, but sometimes when it was easier for me just to sit in my chair rather than heave myself up to bed, you can imagine that tidying up was never high on my priority list. There was takeaway packaging on the carpet ... you name it, I'd had it delivered. Food deliveries weren't for a special occasion or Saturday-night treats now. It was a regular phone call at any time of the day, whether actually at home or on my way home.

My other friend was with me that night – TV. I'd sit in front of it night after night, a Groundhog Day of overeating; TV dinners forming my staple calorie-uncontrolled diet in addition to TV breakfasts, TV elevenses, TV brunches, TV lunches, TV teas, TV suppers and TV snacks. You get the idea – food and TV.

Another constant was the pain in my joints, with my legs covered in weeping sores and agonising ulcers that never healed. My self-esteem couldn't have got any lower. I had become one of the fattest men in the UK. The scene was of one an archetypical slob's living room in a sitcom, but without the empty cans of beer. It was a scene from my own show, *Man Eating Badly* – my bachelor pad in my own situation tragedy. I was literally eating myself into oblivion day after day, and if the eating didn't kill me, I could only see one other choice.

I sat there wishing I was dead.

It's not every day you get the opportunity to write your autobiography, is it? Where do you start something like this? I'm quite used to the odd interview now, but an entire life story is quite different. Talk about being under pressure! I am well aware that I am not quite an international superstar with millions of adoring fans (yet). I mean, I've always considered myself to be a pretty average bloke really, but my story is rather unique. That uniqueness is the reason you just bought this book ... not because I was in a boy band or because I'm a Hollywood actor or scored goals for England (I'm sure all those will come in time anyway), but because you know who I am and want to know more about how I became so large and how I motivated myself to become Slimmer Charlie.

As a big comedy fan, I started reading one of Frank Skinner's books recently and thought it would give me a few pointers on how to write mine. He starts off by saying if he's thinking about buying a book he'll read the first paragraph in the shop, as this gives a fair indication of what the rest of the book will be like. Hence me getting the girl, killing the baddies and saving the planet. I thought it would be a bit more of a hook than telling you where and when I was born. He

13

also mentions that he gives up reading biographies if he gets to page fifty and the subject of the book is still at school. I'm like that with books too ... jog on to when you are famous! Get to the scandal and the sleeping around with groupies section! I'll make sure to put the story about when Fern Britton came knocking on my dressing room door on page forty-nine.

Not many people had such a remarkable childhood that it is worth dwelling on for three quarters of a book, but I do think that those early years shape you into what you are as an adult. To write this, I did a lot of soul-searching and discovered the above to be true. Other than trying to purposefully skip over the early days, I think if we're going to be spending so much time together then you need to know about my background. Imagine the reviews ... 'Excellent book, but Walduck neglected to tell us anything about when he was young, so no one identified with him.'

So, for the record, I, Charles Ambrose Walduck, was born on 30 August 1968 at Risedale Maternity Hospital in Barrow-in-Furness and weighed in at six pounds and six ounces. The first of three for proud parents Janet and Clifford, I was named after my two grandfathers, Charles Cherry and Ambrose Walduck.

I was born by Caesarean section and I've still got a scar from my birth when the doctor managed to cut my head. I'm sure that didn't help ease the tension. Mum had been pregnant before and had lost her first child during birth and very nearly lost her own life in the process. It's impossible to imagine the loss and the hurt – and so, whilst pregnant with me, it was a very anxious and stressful time for them both. Every day must have been a mixture of emotion and going into C-section must have brought all those memories flooding back to the surface. It must be heart wrenching to have to deal with such things and it takes strong people to survive. I'm proud of them for that. My mum must think about this often and I know in my dark days of feeling low and suicidal it must really upset her.

My brother Steven joined the clan in November 1970 and my sister Jackie completed the line-up in December 1971. Steven is married with two children and now lives in Aberdeen and Jackie has four children and lives not too far away in Ulverston.

We always got along fine apart from the usual sibling rivalry, but there were lots of happy memories of the times we all spent together. Steven was the sporty one, leaving me as the non-sporty one. I couldn't even get my head around those video games where you could play football, tennis and dozens of other sports (but they all managed to be exactly the same game – what was all that about?). So where Steven was into anything that involved fitness, with me in tow we were never going to give the Neville brothers a run for their money in anything other than a beauty contest. I was never the type to play out that much and didn't really have any friends, so most of my playtime was spent indoors with Steven and Jackie or other family members. We were very close in that respect. My mum and dad always made sure we were kept warm and comfortable, extremely well fed and clothed and were given lots of love and affection. Although we were by no means spoiled (Mum and Dad couldn't afford to), I am conscious that I am so very lucky to have had a normal, happy childhood.

At the age of five I started at St James' Infant School. Being born in August, I had only just turned five when I started school and was always the youngest in the class. I didn't take to school well at all. Not that there

15

was anything wrong with the school itself: looking back now, I can see that I was very sensitive to other peoples' thoughts toward me. It sounds mad, but I'd stand in the playground on my own with the fear of rejection making it impossible for me to bond and play like all the other kids were doing. I thought they would look at me and say 'What's he doing here?' 'What right has he to be here?' What if nobody liked me ... what would I do? I don't know what it was, but I've always been a worrier. I was just too nervous in that situation. I've often put this down to the anguish that Mum was going through when she was carrying me because of her last experience of pregnancy. It's like I took on board those feelings she must have had and they became part of my personality. Once I was on a bus with my mum and was convinced she hadn't paid my fare. I felt uncomfortable for the whole journey, thinking we'd get thrown off, thinking the worst, squirming all the way home. As we were getting off the bus, I asked the driver if she'd paid, just to make sure. Of course she had and there'd been no reason to worry. Try telling me that, though.

It was maybe around this age that I used to wet the bed. Some of the symptoms for this are said to be worry and stress, although some would argue that a five year old shouldn't have any stress or worry in their life. I agree. It shouldn't have been there, but for whatever reason, it was. Bedwetting is also a very common thing in kids and there's always a need to label something or find a reason when sometimes there isn't one. Sometimes things just happen 'because' and there is no other explanation. I used to worry *because*; I used to wet the bed *because*. And that's it. I used to hate having to lie there waiting for Mum to come and change the sheets. I still feel embarrassed and guilty when I think back to those nights of lying in a wet bed like it was my fault and I'd done wrong and I was causing upset. If I'd known it was a common thing, I probably still would have worried.

These feelings of not fitting in and not having a right to be there stayed with me throughout my life and still remain with me now. I've always been painfully shy – it's odd, because some of the things I've done in my life, you'd expect me to be very extrovert. It's just how I am. I know people who are great public speakers and teachers and they'll admit to being shy too. It's an odd contradiction that people find difficult to believe. I suppose it's a bit like taking on a role, pretending, putting on an act and having that role or mask to hide behind.

Because of my sensitivity, I often felt let down quite a bit as a youngster too. There was one day I was in the park with my dad, who'd just bought me a lovely new kite to fly. In no time at all it got tangled up in some railings and it was game over for the kite. I was gutted. I just expected my dad to take me to buy another one, but it wasn't to be. Whether it was because times were tough or simply to teach me the value of things, I learnt the hard way from occasions such as these.

Dad, like so many others in Barrow, worked at the shipyard and strikes were not unusual. There would always be ups and downs, especially in great industries like mining and shipbuilding, where management and unions clashed on a regular basis and the workers downed tools and walked. We grew up quite used to struggling to get by from time to time, but no matter how difficult things were, we never ever went hungry.

The only proper good memory I have from school is school dinners. I loved them! The dinner ladies would always give extra to the chubby kids. And being one of the chubbies, I would always get extra. Result! I also think they felt a bit sorry for me as I was quite the Billy-no-mates, and of course, I was never going to refuse seconds. Or thirds, if they were asking. Thinking about it now, it was misplaced kindness, but what's done is done. With their help, I managed to invent childhood obesity, becoming a chunky child long before it became popular. In the school's defence, it wasn't that the food was unhealthy, same with the food I had at home. It was just that I was starting to eat it all in such large quantities.

It was common knowledge that any waste from the school dinners would get piled up and turned into pigswill – and oh how I envied those pigs. Other than getting slaughtered and ending up in sandwiches, they were pretty much sorted.

Mum used to give us ten pence spending money each week on a Monday and again on a Friday and I would spend mine on crisps and sweets. Mum never allowed any of us to have chewing gum, because she said it would wrap around our throats and kill us. I remember once picking some chewing gum up off the pavement and eating it, just to see what it was like and if it was as dangerous as I'd been led to believe, although, in this instance, I reckon the germs posed a bigger threat to my health than the actual chewing gum did. It quite put me off chewing gum. Up until I dared to try it again years later, I thought it all tasted like cigarettes and dirt. It was a nice surprise.

My desire for food of any type became so strong I would do almost anything to get it. Eating started to get its claws into me, much like any other addict, but I was always in check with my morals: I'd never steal, take anything without paying and would never eat the scraps off other people's plates. I remember seeing someone in the school canteen passing from table to table finishing off what people had left and I felt embarrassed for him. For me to be young and this interested in food wasn't right. I know it is always encouraging to see kids with a healthy appetite, but mine went that bit further, crossing the line to become an unhealthy one. It was really all I thought about.

I had one friend called Mark when I was around ten years old. I went to his house after school once and his mum made us crinkle-cut oven chips and burgers for dinner. It was the first time I'd tasted oven chips and they were out of this world. We watched *Superman* on TV and I couldn't wait to get back home and spread the word. Mums always ask you what you had when you go out to tea and my mum was no different. She was amazed that people bought frozen chips – in our house it was always a sack of potatoes, done the traditional way. Oven chips may have been the latest fad, but crinkle-cut ones were the future. I knew because I'd seen it. Who needed to go to the trouble of peeling and slicing a potato anymore? Sure enough, the next question to come from me was, 'Can we have crinkle-cut oven chips?' Mum was reluctant to follow the new ways, but she compromised and bought a crinkle chip cutter instead. All the kids were singing 'Hope it's chips, it's chips' in the tune of 'Que Sera, Sera' from the oven chips TV advert, and Crispy Pancakes were all the rage. In short, these were good times to have an oven and a freezer and I didn't want us to get left behind. Who needs chip pan fires when you just need to rip a bag open and bang them on an oven tray?

When we had guests for dinner or tea, I noticed their portions would be much bigger than ours. What was that about, I pondered? It didn't seem fair.

'It's polite,' Mum would say. 'Guests should get the largest portions.'

Hmm ... Sadly, I soon realised that when I sat down to dinner at other people's houses and looked down at my meagre portion, not everyone thought like my mum. Some people have no manners! When we visited my nana and granddad (Dad's parents) they always were polite when it came to dishing out the grub. Nana would spoil us with all the usual treats that grandparents have specially tucked away for their grandchildren. They lived around eight miles away and we would all go quite regularly to see them. Families don't seem to spend enough time visiting each other these days, unless they have to or want to borrow a lawnmower. Nana Lillian was a fantastic cook and I have amazing memories of Granddad Ambrose, who was a really special man – one of those types you look up to and respect and want to be in their company.

Sometimes we'd visit them at night and would drive over with us three dressed in our pyjamas. It was a great adventure. If you've got kids, you'll know how excited they get if you ever do a mad pyjamas outing ... we giggled and snuggled all the way there.

Nothing could beat Christmas dinner at their house; the food was to die for. Unfortunately, Nana was always busy in the kitchen half the day preparing, so by the time she was ready to sit down for hers (serving herself last) we'd be cleaning our plates ready of seconds. She was great – always making sure everyone was happy and fed.

Jackie and Steven were never quite as interested in Christmas, but to me it was sheer magic. I would wake up and ask 'Has he been?' I always knew it was Mum and Dad filling the stockings up rather than Santa, because my Spock-like mind couldn't cope with the concept of his existence. But what the hell – if he (they) were going to bring me a bag of chocolate then I was happy to 'believe'. Our day would start with opening presents in the morning, then getting ready for our trip to Nana's, usually after sampling some of my Christmas goodies first, just as an appetiser.

She was never the tidiest person in the world. Once, she stood surveying the living room and said, 'Oh dear the house is a bit untidy.'

'Yes. I can see that,' I replied, and got a clip round the ear for my trouble! I can laugh about it now, but at the time I was only agreeing with her. I mean, my delivery could have been a lot more sarcastic, if that's what I was going for. I'll not be doing that again in a hurry, I can tell you. Hell hath no fury like a woman when you agree that her house is a mess.

During one of our Christmas dinners there, a sprout flew from Nana's plate when she was eating and Dad said, 'Don't worry, mother. You'll find it next year when you clean up.' (This is one of those stories that my mum and dad always reminisce about fondly. As a family, humour has always played a big part in our lives with us all trying to outdo each other – even now. Dad's jokes are typical dad jokes, and now that I've got the opportunity to put them in black and white, they really are terrible.)

Anyway, we would be at bursting point after dinner and Nana would always ask if we wanted more. Seriously though, I always did have seconds, and by the time we'd had pudding, I was lucky if I could move. It wasn't easy having eyes as big as my belly.

Even though it was Christmas, the alarm bells should have been ringing by now: there was a bit of a problem. It was like a compulsion, no plate could be left until it was empty, no offer of more could be refused. Maybe it's easier to think of it all as a one off until it becomes blatantly obvious that it isn't. And that's usually when the problem is too late.

I used to love the smell of the turkey cooking on Christmas Day. Just like when Mum used to bake her own bread, it's one of those aromas that captivate you – a real Bisto Kid moment (for those old enough to remember). We'd laugh at all those people who'd talk about turkey lasting for weeks and weeks – if we'd had any left on Boxing Day it would have been a miracle.

I loved family celebrations. Other people would visit us too, so there was always some sort of socialising going on. I liked that we were surrounded by family. It was never overbearing – we were a family who actually enjoyed being in each other's company and didn't just do it because we thought we had to.

Birthday parties were such special occasions for me as well. I used to get so excited and wound up knowing there was a party about to start. I loved the build-up: the busyness in the kitchen, the cooking smells, the table being set, the party games being prepared ... the feeling was incredible. All our family and friends would be invited and Mum would put on an enormous spread with all sorts of children's party food. It was like heaven: cakes, sandwiches, pies, sausage rolls, jellies and trifle would all be laid out ready for us to tuck in. It was like being on set of the latest 'Mum's gone to Iceland' advert. Naturally, I would be the last to leave the table and I'd still be on savouries when everyone else was on the cakes and trifle.

After the highs of parties, there always came a big low for me. I never wanted them to end. I'd always want to carry on playing games and hated it when the other children had to leave. I just couldn't let go. At the end of one birthday party, I was so upset when it was time for the children to go home, I pleaded for more games of pass the parcel – even though that meant wrapping up one of the gifts I had been given that day. Whatever it took, I'd do it.

My birthdays generally ended the same way: I'd go to bed and cry myself to sleep, sad that the day had ended and then I'd be left with a bad memory of it ending rather than a good one of it having taken place. It was the same at Christmas. It was difficult to deal with as no one really seemed to understand the anxiety and then depression it caused. I felt so frantic when I knew something was drawing to a close, my brain going into overdrive to think of ways to prolong it. This is something else that has followed me throughout my life, whether it was the end of a holiday, the end of a night out or simply the end of having a nice day. It didn't matter. It started to feel like there was a constant low that the festivities lifted for a bit. That's why I didn't want them to end. No one else seemed to go through this. Sure, others didn't like parties ending, but to me it felt a lot more than just a party ending: the entire mood would have to come back down to normality, the whole house transformed back and I found it so difficult to readjust.

On Tuesdays, my Auntie Carol would come round in the evening and my dad would go off to watch Barrow playing football. With Dad out the house it meant only one thing – riot time! Like all kids, we'd take full advantage of the ruling hand being out for a couple of hours. Mum would use the 'Wait 'til your dad gets home' card and we'd use the 'Make sure to get round

Mum before Dad gets home' card. It was all pure entertainment, really. With Auntie Carol there and my dad out, it was just our way of keeping the laughs going. All kids have a bit of a mess on when they know they can get away with it. Order was usually restored by the time he returned from the footy, apart from the time I came out with, 'Dad's gone. Let's start messing around!' then legged it downstairs, burst into the living room ... to find Dad still at home. Then the ruling hand gave me a smacked arse. I still maintain to this day that I knew he was there and I was just having a laugh. Did anyone believe me? No one believed me when the cat knocked the glass fish off the TV either. That's adults for you.

My Auntie Elaine (not a real auntie – but sort of related) would come for lunch on Wednesdays. She was a big lady with a big heart and I just loved listening to tales about her life. She'd tell us about buying Easter eggs and how she would always end up eating them before giving them as gifts. Same with selection boxes at Christmas. She'd have to go out and buy them again and would end up eating the second lot as well. A lady after my own heart! And embarrassingly, I always told her that one day I would marry her. I always felt comfortable in her company and she certainly knows how to make me squirm ... every time I see her now, she reminds me of my promise.

Moving swiftly on, Nana and Granddad would also visit on a Wednesday and Mum would make one of my favourites – Cheese and Onion Pie and Egg and Bacon Pie (or quiche to you and me), chips, beans, and pudding too. And no, not all on the same plate. I may have liked eating, but I'm not mad.

The big table would go up and I would be in my element. How I loved Wednesdays – the smell of my mum's cooking and Granddad's roll ups – happy family days. We would sit and watch TV in the evening, and without fail, just before *This Is Your Life* came on, Auntie Elaine would say 'Janet, go and get your dress on!' to Mum. It became a tradition. I would always sneak off and come back with my hair slicked down, with a hairbrush for a microphone, and tell my mum 'Tonight, Janet Walduck ... this is *your* life!' To make it more authentic I'd taped the theme tune to the show on one of those cassette recorders where you'd set the microphone up next to the speaker in complete silence. I always fancied being a TV presenter or something like that. I loved performing to an audience. It was something that brought me out of my shell and I felt really comfortable doing it.

Saturday was our turn to visit Auntie Carol. My dad would go to the football match and afterwards we would all walk home together. Another great thing about Saturdays was that for tea we always had party food: sandwiches, cakes (remember when Fondant Fancies were a proper size and not just gone in a bite like they are now?), pork pies, trifle, jelly, sausage rolls ... the kind of food that made my whole face light up! It was the sort of treat I never tired of one single bit – a party every week. One Saturday we were walking there when an ambulance went screeching past us and up the road from where we had just come. Unknown to us, as we were having a leisurely stroll, Steven had been knocked off his bike by a car. Someone must have seen it and phoned for help immediately. It turned out he was OK, but the consequence was that we had sausage, mash and gravy because there hadn't been time to prepare the usual. I wasn't at all happy about missing out on the weekly treat. For such a dramatic day in our life and one that was traumatic for us all, my memory of it is still of the food I missed out on.

I was never that religious, but I used to pray on Sunday mornings. For rain. You see, our Sundays were reserved for Dad taking us out for walks and I'd try almost anything, other than breaking one of my own legs, to get out of it. It was like having one of The Proclaimers as a parent (both of them as parents would have been plain weird). He was never one to do things by half, my dad – a walk was a loose term for a trek in his language. To be fair, I did eventually enjoy the walks and it was great to have the sense of achievement at the end of it. Back at home, Dad would get a shoelace out and measure on the map how far we had walked and I'd be like Roy Scheider in *Jaws*, giving it, 'Dad, you're gonna need a bigger lace.'

One day we managed to walk twenty miles. See what I mean about a trek? On New Year's Day we would always walk over to Granddad's house to let the New Year in. He'd drive us back though. In those days it was called exercise and fresh air, but today it would be child abuse, I'm sure. You can't put kids through stuff like that these days! It was like trying out for the army. Somehow, Steven and Jackie used to get out of going. I can't even remember how, all I know is there can't be any justice in the world. The walks became known as the Sunday Club and there were fourteen of us at one point. You know, with all the camaraderie that went with trekking round the countryside, it did give me a great sense of belonging, to be out there and be a part of something. It was a bond to share that the others didn't have with my dad.

While all that was going on, Mum would be at home preparing our meal and the best part of the day was when we were on the home stretch. There was always a great sense of security from being out doing the manly pursuits to coming home to the warmth and a nice, hearty meal. Mum's Sunday roast dinners were heavenly and she'd never vandalise it by using instant gravy either – it was all done the traditional way. There's nothing worse than doing most of something well and then spoiling it all at the last hurdle. Like when you go for a pub meal and have lovely bangers and onion gravy on a bed of Smash. Makes me shiver just thinking about it.

Jackie and I used to have to do the washing up afterwards – yet another chore Steven got out of. He once 'accidentally' broke a plate and wasn't trusted to do the dishes ever again. Wish I'd thought of that first. We'd always argue about who would wash and who would dry. It got to the point where we'd ask weeks in advance so we could get one over each other by reserving which we wanted to do.

Sunday evenings would drag and drag on. What was it with them? It was miserable – the thought of school the next day and the end of the weekend. Even now I think Sundays have a strange feel to them. It's like being in limbo, just waiting for the inevitable Monday morning. It was bath and hair wash night as well on a Sunday, just to make things worse. Mum would turn off the TV and put the wireless on instead, as if to make the night drag out even further. It wasn't like she used to have the Sunday Chart Show on either, but usually something kids found boring. It was a case of riding out the boredom until supper time at eight o'clock. There would be a piece of cake or pie and sandwiches – never crisps though (I'll tell you why later). It was nice to round the week off with a bit of sweet 'n' savoury.

I know I used 'abuse' earlier as a tongue-in-cheek description, but when you're young, anything you don't want to do feels like torture. Even down to having a nice, hot bath, something too many of us take for granted. Sounds mad thinking about it now. It wasn't that long before my time when it was tin baths in front of the fire. Now that would have been something to complain about!

You'll be starting to see the pattern emerging. My life has always been ruled by food. I can make the odd joke about it here and there but actually sitting down and writing about it makes it all the more poignant. People who used to play out all the time as kids will have things like the smell of freshly cut grass to remind them of an endless summer holiday, or the sounds of running water if they found a river to play by. All I seem to have is the smell of some food in the oven or the sound something made as it was cooking. If I'd been around, I couldn't tell you where I was when Kennedy got shot, but I'd be able to tell you what food I was eating in minute detail. Should I have known there was a problem early on? Should others have spotted it? Was it anyone's fault? I have no idea. I'd always perceived people with problems and addictions later in life as people who probably didn't have the best upbringing, with a troubled childhood and dysfunctional family. I had none of that.

But then there are always the little signs ... having no real friends, no real bonds with other kids my age, not playing out, being very sensitive, not wanting things to end and having to compulsively eat to the point of being sick rather than let something go to waste. It's almost like food was my friend and the friendship began to develop from an early age. Most childhood friendships are on and off with fallings out over the years. Not this one. It flourished.

When Dad was on night shift we would all sit at the table for breakfast and have cereal and toast on the morning. I bet it felt good to come back from doing hard graft to the warmth of his family and somewhere to rest his weary bones. Mum would tell him about what she had watched on TV the night before and would go into the entire plot of films and programmes to the point where it was like we'd all watched them. I just loved listening to everything she had to say. Dad would then head off to bed and we would get ready for school. It wouldn't be long before Dad would stomp back downstairs to tell us to keep the noise down. Even with the best intentions, it's difficult to get three kids ready for school in silence. You should have heard the din when Mum and Steven used to do exercise along with Mad Lizzy on *TV-am*. All hope of him getting off to sleep before we'd left the house was lost.

I looked forward to Friday mornings because we'd sit down to a cooked breakfast. I mean ... sausages, bacon, eggs, mushrooms, hash browns, beans, tomatoes ... tea, toast ... there is no finer way to start your day. Or end it. Being woken up by the smell of it all sizzling away in a pan beats any alarm clock. Fridays had a real sense of occasion, like we were celebrating the last day of a working week, and Mum would lay the table the night before in preparation.

You always know you are growing up when you get your own front door key. It was a big deal for me – one of the perks of being the eldest child, and it gave me a fantastic sense of trust. It was Mum and Dad recognising that I was becoming responsible, rather than arranging for someone to come round. With them no longer being at home on a Friday when we got home from school (Dad was at work and Mum used to go shopping), just like the American sitcom, I was *Charles in Charge* for the night.

The television was always on when I opened the door with my shiny new key on Fridays. It was reassuring in a way, but a bit eerie in others as I'd always expect someone to be in. Mum made our tea for us and left it on plates in the kitchen before they went out, so there wasn't any faffing on to be done. I may have been the responsible one, but there was no way I was going to start making tea when I got home. I wasn't *that* responsible! I have a particular aversion to anyone touching my food so there was a bit of trial and error in respect of the food being left out, until Mum started to put nametags on our plates (mine was easy to spot anyway as it was always the largest of the three). We all felt grown up being left to our own devices. I mean, we could watch whatever we wanted on TV – but in those days there were only three channels.

Twice a year we would go to visit my Gran down in Devon and make a real holiday of it. Two weeks in the summer in Torquay was something to look forward to, I can tell you. Granddad Charles died when I was only three years old and my only memory of him is that he had a bed downstairs. According to Mum, he was so proud that I was named after him, and although he was known as Charlie, my mum hates me being called Charlie. I take it it's too late to change the title of this book. Woe betides anyone who'd ring up asking for me by that name. There was 'no one called Charlie here'. Mums are always protective of your first name, aren't they? They never shorten it.

Unfortunately, Gran was not in the same league as Nana when it came to cooking. It was the downside to spending two weeks there, but you had to just grin and bear it. Not that her cooking was *terrible*, just not as good as. Foodies recognise these things, you know. After my granddad passed away it was just Gran and Auntie Margaret, my mum's sister. Auntie Margaret had a great sense of silly humour and I always got on really well with her. She was never ashamed of me when I became bigger (hate to spoil the rest of the book for you by dropping that one in). Ever. With just seeing each other twice a year, she'd probably have noticed the weight gain more than others, but she never commented and it never affected our relationship. She was ace and I know she would have been proud of me for doing what I've done.

Devon was such a relaxed place to spend summer. Dad especially loved Gran and Margaret's house because they had a back garden; something we never had at home, and I often felt for him, not having one. He grew all sorts of fruit and vegetables in theirs and really enjoyed having a part-time hobby. They had apple and cherry trees, but Dad would warn me:

'Don't go eating all the fruit. It's not like it grows on trees, you know.'

'If they fall on the ground, then they have to be eaten,' replied Charlie 'tree shaker' Walduck innocently.

I'd still munch the fruit, but I was always wondering if pork pie trees would ever grow.

They moved up to Barrow in 1979, to a council house on Walney Island. We drove down to Torquay to collect them to bring them to their new life and I remember wishing so hard it was us moving to Devon and not the other way round. It was such a shame to miss out on those holidays, but at least it meant that Gran and Auntie Margaret were closer to us, so we gained in other ways. I would often stay overnight at their house without Jackie and Steven and they would spoil me so much with treats galore. Happy days!

With nowhere to go for our summer holidays we started to go on camping trips. Why does everyone set off with such a romantic vision of idyllic bliss? Camping, roughing it, living off the land, the fresh air, the countryside, the great outdoors ... however you dress it up, it just means no comfort, no central heating, wind blowing through the tent and tins of beans cooked on a camping stove. Fresh air – go on, I'll give you that one. I'm more of a great indoors type though. Mum and Dad bought us a big house tent, which should have had separate rooms, but somehow we never bothered partitioning it off, so we ended up in the huge open-plan tent together. I have to admit (sorry, Mum and Dad) that I hated it. Cornflakes with warm milk, flies swarming around the food and the rain dripping in the tent all night, and on top of all that – no toilet. Maybe I'm not getting my point across here, but *I didn't take to camping at all*. Not one bit. I vividly remember Mum being terrified that a sheep was going to come into the tent and pounce on her. I mean, this was her idea, and even she was freaking out about gangs of delinquent livestock on the loose. We should have sent Gran and Auntie Margaret a postcard saying 'Wish you were still in Devon.'

I also hated having to get undressed in front of everyone. Perhaps even at this stage of my life I was aware of my body, and I'd started to grow up and enter puberty. Those days of being a kid and running around with nothing on without shame were gone. Yes, we're all the same underneath, but that's no reason to turn the place into a nudist camp. We would go swimming loads when we were roughing it and I would hide behind the bushes to get undressed before hoofing it to the edge and jumping straight in. Dad used to tell me to stop worrying about it and to let it all hang out, but that was not me at all. Some people can do things like that and not care, but I care, so I can't. It gave me a sense of vulnerability that I didn't like – whether it was my immediate family who I was with or not, it didn't matter. I was always first into the water and last out. Once I was in, I loved swimming and would spend hours in the water – lakes, rivers, the sea, anywhere. The initial hit of cold water then the freedom of being able to swim and be part of nature ... it's enough to make it sound like I enjoyed outdoor pursuits, so I'll not big it up too much. There was the walking and picnics through the day that were nice too, but still ... it wasn't home and there was never any comfort.

My Auntie Doreen and Uncle Keith were also into camping and we would often all go together, although they were far more professional than us. However, that didn't stop their tent blowing away one night. It just goes to show, you can be prepared, head to toe in all the latest gear, be the next Bear Grylls even, but it can still go wrong. I wished ours would blow away too. I was never that lucky.

In the evenings, Mum and Dad would go to the local pub and we would sit outside. I know that sounds terrible because Mum and Dad were never big pub goers. In fact, Dad would brew his own lager and they would rather have a couple of drinks at home. When camping though, they would go to the local pub (maybe they needed some time alone, or to numb the pain). While they were in, Mum would keep coming out with supplies of pop and crisps and to make sure we were alright. And now your brain has just flagged up the word 'crisps' from earlier. Top marks if you were paying attention. Dad hated us having crisps for three reasons: the crunching sound they made (yes, really), they were expensive, and they would make us fat. He was at least right on the last point. Up until the age of twenty-six, I always sucked on my crisps so they wouldn't make a noise.

Imprinted on my mind is a photo of us all standing outside the tent on one of these expeditions, and I'm there, big boobs, moobs if you will, even at the age of thirteen. Looking at that photo, I could see what other people saw and I didn't like it. I felt embarrassed to realise that's what people saw and imagined what they'd be thinking. It's a horrible, sinking feeling.

I guess I was a little frightened of my dad. Dads are always the main 'enforcer' in the traditional role of family life, so I think everyone has been a bit wary of their dad at some point. If we were ever too naughty we would be sent to bed early, which carried an even worse punishment with it – missing out on supper! Dad could look quite stern at times and that look was generally enough to put a stop to whatever bad behaviour was going on. Dads are good at that. There must be a book somewhere with dad rules, regulations and advice on the right look for every occasion: *How to Stop your Children Fighting with Facial Expression Only ... How to Lighten the Mood by Doing Something Silly, Pretending to Trip Over or by Facial Expression Only.* Behind the sometimes-stern expression there was a heart of gold and we could always rely on him if we needed anything. That's what dads are for and they all know this regardless of whether they have the mythical *Dad Rule Book* or not.

34

At the age of eleven, I started at Alfred Barrow Secondary School, and to get there and back I had to walk through Barrow town centre, passing lovely cafes and pie shops along the way.

I enjoyed going to secondary school, though it was always marred by my shyness. I would have loved to get involved in the drama groups and be a bit more active, but with my lack of confidence and self-esteem, my courage always deserted me and I was left looking on and dreaming of what might have been. Maybe playing the Lion in *The Wizard of Oz* would have been fitting.

So with any acting aspirations being a non-starter, I had no idea what I wanted to do with my life. I was never one of those who knew as soon as they were born what they wanted to do and stuck to it. Thank God. At one point, I joined a club along with some friends called the FTG (the Furness Transport Group), who had an old double-decker bus that they would take to bus rallies and carnivals. I had no idea bus rallies even existed until then. It was great fun. And one thing you may have noticed is that I joined *with some friends* ... I wasn't Charlie-no-mates anymore.

Most of the kids in the group were those who'd be labelled as nerds these days. We were not exactly cool, being a member of a bus group, in the eyes of others anyway, but to me it was great because we travelled around the country in an old double-decker bus.

For a short time I wanted to be a bus conductor. Don't know why, really. They got to stand around on buses and it probably seemed a bit cool at the time. If cool is the right word. But they were being phased out and when I thought about being a bus driver instead, to keep the bus theme going, I thought no way could I do that because I couldn't drive. Even at twelve years old, the famous self-doubt held me back. Why would I tell myself I couldn't drive? My voice hadn't even broken and I was still at school. It was quite obvious that I couldn't drive, but it was like this inner-me would always drag me back to reality once a dream was hatched; like it was poised with a pin ready to burst any bubble.

If watching TV and, well, it could have been anything really – a singer in a band, someone playing football, a magician – if anyone came on who could do something, I'd get 'You couldn't do that,' 'They wouldn't want you,' and 'You're incapable of that' from Mum and Dad. It's never nice for any child to hear a parent have such un-great expectations and this is something that does affect kids later in life. It was like being conditioned and it surfaces any time I feel great and positive; it's always there in the background to repress those feelings of having and worth. It had a massive impact on my life, being brought down in such a way. If they knew what they were doing, they'd have stopped. Rather than it being a malicious thing, I think it was all largely because of Mum's background. Her mum worked in service at a stately home as a maid and her dad was the groundsman, so all that 'knowing your place in life' attitude stemmed from that.

It's no wonder there are so many messed-up people in the world because parents have always thrown such off-the-cuff comments at their kids, always put them down through what they'd call 'only having a laugh', and those are the things kids take with them into adulthood. Stop doing it! I was always a sensitive lad, always will be ... maybe I took it all too much to heart. I know it had an impact on my confidence. I've never pushed myself career-wise. I'm just not that type. Steven is successful in life and Jackie has so much confidence. How are they so different? How didn't they turn out the same as me? Well, I just don't know. Maybe it all rubbed off on me because I'm the more sensitive. I know the kind of comments that were dished out would just go over Steven and Jackie's heads. Maybe there is no proper explanation, no real reason other than we're all different; no two people are the same.

In those days, career aspirations began with going on a YTS (Youth Training Scheme for those of you under thirty-five) and getting a trade. My dad used to always come out with that one, as I'm sure every other dad in the country did. 'You've got to get yourself a trade' was used by dads in a time when there was trade and industry in the country. Nowadays everyone is looking for careers in telecoms and IT and the jobs for life in industry that employed entire communities are a thing of the past. I used to tell Dad it was never going to happen. I wasn't going to be a shipbuilder. I may have looked for a job doing admin in the site office, but there weren't any jobs in that side of the industry.

Dad was made redundant in the early 1980s and

bought a static caravan with his redundancy pay. It was a nice thing to do for the family and it meant that our weekends and holidays were sorted for life. I loved it! I'd spend ages swimming when we were there – it's a wonder I didn't grow gills. I was like Bobby Ewing in *The Man from Atlantis*.

During the odd times when I was on dry land, I started helping out around the camp, doing any odd jobs and as a result of socialising, slowly but surely, I began to emerge from my shell (pardon the marine-based pun).

On Sunday afternoons they would have a kids' talent show and every week I would get on stage and tell some jokes. I enjoyed it and, for some reason, with a microphone in my hand I could be a different person. It was if someone had given me a free pass to have a life. It was just like doing the Eamonn Andrews impression at home with the hairbrush; I could be someone else as long as I had something to hide behind. Typically, nobody laughed. I didn't think I was that bad if I'm honest. Talk about a tough crowd! I think I was just ahead of my time. Dad was the only one who laughed and quickly my catchphrase became 'Thanks, Dad.' At least we enjoyed ourselves. Maybe having the king of the bad jokes laughing at mine was a sign of something.

One afternoon I was asked if I fancied calling some bingo numbers for the caravan owners. I was only around fifteen years old and this was my first bingo gig. Boy, was I amazing. I know I'm being a bit coy about it all, but I was out of this world – I took to it like a (Wal)duck to water. It all seemed to come naturally to me, like I already knew what I was supposed to do, like I was answering to my calling. At school one day afterwards, I told the careers adviser that I wanted to be a professional bingo caller. I can't remember exactly what the response was, but I doubt there have been many others with that career path since. It would be great to know I was his success story that he told other pupils about once I'd 'made it'. 'Oh yeah. Charlie Walduck? He said he liked numbers and the entertainment industry so I told him to be a bingo caller. It's all down to me.'

I tried my hand at so many other jobs at the caravan park: I was a DJ, glass collector, cleaner and barman extraordinaire! Any job that cropped up I'd give it a go. It gave me so much confidence and independence. I wasn't a shy kid anymore. Of course, I was deep down, but you wouldn't think it on the outside. It got to the point where Mum and Dad used to leave me behind on a Sunday evening and return to Barrow. Being sixteen years of age with a caravan all to myself was a stomach-churner of excitement. And a stomach filler, as it happened. It was such a buzz to be alone there with the adventure of fending for myself. I think it was more because I knew it was short-lived freedom and I could return to normality, rather than being stuck for real in an adult life, that felt so good. A taster was all I wanted.

One evening, just after I'd waved goodbye to Mum and Dad and watched the car disappear out of view, and despite the fact I had just eaten a big meal, I decided to cook myself some beef burgers. It was a craving I couldn't resist. They were there and so was I. Out came the frying pan, the gas was cranked up, the oil was sizzling and I was happily cooking away when the caravan door opened. To my horror Mum and Dad had turned back because they had forgotten something. My mum immediately demanded to know what I was cooking and why. I was so embarrassed; I could have died on the spot. I stammered something about making the burgers for my supper so I wouldn't have to mess on when I returned from the club. To this day I am not sure if they believed me and they would have been right not to. See, for me it was never a case of having my own space to throw wild parties and get drunk. A bit of freedom was freedom to indulge in my one and only vice.

Also, round about this time, I'd lost most of my puppy fat and for a while I was quite slender; something else short-lived. Working at the holiday camp during the summer months meant I was earning real money and not relying on pocket money handouts. As it was *my* hard-earned money, I could spend it how I liked and on what I liked: food. Glorious food, in fact. As the weekends rolled on, so did the pounds I was gaining. The money literally was in one hand and out the other. The holiday camp was fine because they'd pay me and I'd spend it all there. At one point, Steven had a job there and so did my dad. When we first got the caravan we used to hire it out when we weren't there so that we could pay the ground rent, but then we made a pact to all get jobs so we wouldn't have to do this. We'd do odd jobs here and there and it paid our way. Dad used to cut the grass and it all went into the Caravan Savings Fund and meant we could spend all of our summer there. It was a great way to live and it taught me about having to earn money to pay your way in life.

One day when I was about fifteen, back home in Barrow, I remember walking out of the shop on Bath Street with a bag of freshly made pork pies tucked under my arm, straight past Granddad. I was oblivious. I felt ashamed of myself and always used to recall it in my mind to punish myself. There have been plenty of moments in my life like that where you'd assume it would have encouraged me to change my ways out of guilt alone. If I could have I probably would have, but addicts need a bit more than that to 'cure' them. It made me feel bad – it didn't kill me. I could brush it aside. He'd seen me, that much I knew. It was never mentioned and it took me ages to get over the embarrassment of it. Later in life, my dad told me he'd seen me coming out of the same shop armed with pies. It was really distressing because every time I was out of their company he thought I was off somewhere eating. A lot of the time I was, but not always.

Time was running out. Weekend holiday camp work wasn't ideal and Dad had the thumbscrews on me to get a trade and so, like everyone else in school, I applied for an apprenticeship at the shipyard. I never got it and I was not surprised one bit. Thank God. I just wasn't very good at anything practical or mechanical; it wasn't my thing at all. Without any work to go into, I ended up at sixth form college doing some further O levels. It's always been the norm for kids to do that when they are undecided and I bet it has also always been a time for widespread panic amongst parents. I was always pretty sure I'd end up doing *something*, I just didn't know what. It wasn't that I was lazy – I literally hadn't been enthused enough by anything to want to do it as a job for the rest of my life. I only had one friend there called John, but more so because we were outcasts rather than mates as such. We just spoke to each other because neither of us had any friends. It wasn't that enjoyable and I didn't get up to much or make any lasting friendships. It was just a case of walking there on a morning, doing my classes and walking back.

Dad would worry that we would get up to no good as we got older. Drinking, smoking or glue sniffing were the pastimes for many a wayward teenager back then, but it never appealed to me. Even if it did, there was no one to do it with. The closest I ever came to alcohol was walking home one night from sixth form past a drunk who threw a glass of beer over me – just my luck! No idea why anyone would want to do that and I doubt he even knew he'd done it. But he had, and it was me that the bastard did it to. I got home and went straight to the bathroom to put loads of Mum's perfume on to hide the smell of beer. I'd have hated for them to think I'd been out boozing. Satisfied I'd got rid of the smell, I came downstairs without mentioning it at all. I got a few dodgy looks from my dad that night, I can tell you. I think he was suspicious for a completely different reason, although never said anything.

Just before my seventeenth birthday was quite a bad time for us. Dad had a stroke and a heart attack and was in hospital for a while. When he was cutting the grass at the caravan park and used to come into the caravan panting quite badly. He went to the doctor and was told that he was allergic to grass. It wasn't long after that he was taken to hospital after having a mild stroke and was then told that he'd also had a heart attack. He was in hospital for a while and Uncle Keith came to the caravan to help keep us in order because we were a bit wild at the time and Mum found it difficult to cope. Not that many people visited Dad in hospital. I know us kids didn't go and when he was eventually let back home he seemed different in a way. It was only afterwards that I found out he'd been in a bad way and it was touch and go whether he'd pull through. He still gets confused with his words now. I'm not sure medically how to term it all, but it affected the side of the brain that deals with speech rather than the side that can paralyse. It took him a good few months to recover and, once he did, he worked at a restaurant one day a week rather than at the caravan park.

After a couple of years at sixth form college I was still none the wiser about what I wanted to do with my life. To make things worse, I was heading towards page fifty of my memoir and was still at school. I don't know what's worse. I mean, I could easily skip a few years in the memoir, but finding a proper job always takes time. I had a huge interest in what I saw as 'the entertainment industry', though any possibility of a career in this seemed slimmer than Keira Knightley on hunger strike.

There was one more problem as well. I was getting fatter and fatter because of my other huge interest. Dad had noticed and, whilst he weighed in at around nineteen stone himself, told me he thought I'd be as big as him by the time I was eighteen. Sadly, he was right. In fact, I weighed more than he did by that age. I only had myself to blame; I was out of control and desperately in need of help. Overeating has never been recognised as a serious problem or an addiction though. Only in recent years has childhood obesity been flagged up. And that's mostly down to Jamie Oliver, rather than the government initiating anything. Until then kids either got ridiculed and turned into fat adults and ridiculed further, or they were 'normal'. By spending all my money on food I was just like any alcoholic or junkie, experiencing the exact same dependence, but without any assistance to kick my drug habit.

With summer over, I started a BTEC Business Studies

course at Barrow College. I got comments such as 'By the time you finish, you'll be the oldest student in the country' from my dad. He should have known by now what comments like this did to me. It just wasn't funny at all. I had aspirations that had been quashed and I didn't think it worth telling my parents that I wanted to be a performer of some sort because I knew the reaction I'd get. It was sad that I felt that way.

On my first day I stood there in that hall as a nervous, frightened, overweight teenager. It was a bewildering experience being there amongst a sea of strangers, all seemingly with a purpose, knowing what they were doing, where they were going, and then there was me: static. Where I was supposed to fit in amongst all this was anyone's guess. What was Charles Walduck doing in a place like this? What did *he* think he was doing? I was engulfed by all the negativity that I always carry round, yet at the same time it was exciting and I somehow managed to feel optimistic about being there. It was a strange contradiction, but the course started, studies got underway, and I met some great people. Some would become close friends over the years. I desperately wanted people like Mark, Scott and Les (three of my fellow students) to like me. I wanted to be part of the group and I would listen on Fridays as they planned a night out at the weekend and listened on Mondays as they talked about what had gone on at the weekend. I was desperate to be included and I tried to use my humour to endear myself to them. They did grow to like me and I would often meet with Les in the evenings and we would have a walk around Barrow town centre and became good friends.

I had an eighteenth birthday party soon into the course. Naturally, I was too frightened to invite the lads out of fear they'd say no, so it was just the usual crowd present. It was still a great party though. It would have been good to have some new friends there, if only to show I had some. I couldn't have coped with that kind of rejection though, especially early on in a friendship. The thought of asking people I'd just met to commit to *me* ... well, it just filled me with utter dread. There would always be the popular kids in every class and I never was one of them. Years later I told them about the party and they said I should have just invited them and they'd have come along to it. Typical me.

Many nights I'd tell my mum and dad that I was off out to the library as I put my shoes on. But still with earnings from the caravan park, I'd usually have taken money out the bank to go and get pie and chips somewhere in town on an evening. This would be not long after my evening meal, and they didn't have any control over me to stop me. I mean, I wasn't an all-out liar because I did generally go to the library, but it was stopping off for food that was my main motivation for going.

I got involved with the student union and started to become interested in politics and, in 1987, I left home to share a house. It was a tough call and I know it really upset Mum when I left. I dare say it is a massive thing for parents to deal with when their young fly the nest, though this was also a new beginning for me, and a challenging one at that. Rather naively, I assumed Mum was upset because of the expense of me moving out, but she genuinely was upset by it. I got a grant, but, as many of you will know, student grants have never been anything that you can live off.

We shared a house in Church Street and it was good fun. It was an adventure – it always is at first – but it was hugely different from living at home. There was me, Mark, Scott, John and Les, who actually lived next door, but spent most of his time at our place. Times were hard and I couldn't afford much once the rent had been paid.

The first shopping trip we went on together made me realise that they were from more well-off backgrounds because Scott suggested chipping in thirty quid each and I only had a fiver in my pocket to last all week. It made me feel really awkward because if I was expected to put that much money in a week there was no way I'd be able to afford to be a student.

But there was the camaraderie of being in a house with a good bunch of mates, doing silly student things like wiring the TV up to a car battery because we'd heard that meant you didn't need a licence if your parents had one, sitting around with duvets on because we couldn't afford to heat the place and having a small-time gangster as a landlord. Happy days! The week before our first rent payment was due, the landlord came round with four 'heavies' and said, 'Don't forget. Next week the rent is due.' We were stood there at the door telling him we knew.

We were on our best behaviour from the start anyway because we'd heard that he'd nailed someone to the floor for not paying their rent on time. It was a bit weird going to all that trouble to scare a bunch of lads whose only experiences of violence had been watching the wrestling on *World of Sport*. We weren't the maddest student household by any stretch and only had a few nights out here and there. Our main concern was keeping warm at night. That's why we went to the library straight after *Neighbours* until ten o'clock. It was somewhere with free heat and light and somewhere to work from time to time. We were probably the tamest students in history, come to think of it. Personally, I was never the type to grow my hair, wear distressed clothes and tell anyone who'd listen that I'd lost my accent within four days.

I think the most noise we ever made was when I bought a brass band LP from a jumble sale and we played it non-stop. One of the neighbours knocked on the door and told us that he loved brass band music, but not all the time, if you don't mind.

And although money was scarce, I certainly wasn't going to go hungry. I could live as a student, but I was never going to eat like one. I would often go to the chippy just along the street; chips with scraps was my favourite (scraps being bits of batter they'd sieve out of the fryer). And the pie shop on Bath Street was another regular haunt.

Anyone who goes out drinking will have tried out most of the bars in their area and settled on a few they frequent and one they use as a local. It was the same with me, but as I've never drunk nor had any interest in bars, I'd suss out the best places for food in pretty much the same manner: not bad, disgusting, never go back to, good conversation, great grub, clean, good service. And rather than stopping off for a sociably acceptable couple of pints every night of the week, I'd be in the takeaways in town buying food that was just as bad for your health and started becoming less sociably acceptable as my size grew. There's always something guilt-inducing about buying food when you are overweight, you start to recognise the looks from those serving you and can pretty much put money on the conversation being about you when you've left the shop. But basically, living away from home meant that I wasn't being monitored and I could eat all I wanted, all the time.

At lunchtimes I would go up and see Mum and she would make me sandwiches. I'd need be certain that Dad was out because he never liked to see me eat so much. He wasn't being mean; he just didn't want to see me get any bigger, unable to do anything about it.

My flatmates all went home on Fridays and I'd be left rattling around, tidying up, doing the dishes and trying to find things to do to occupy myself. I had a friend called Denise who lived just down the street who I'd go visit and have tea with on a weekend too. She was on our course – there were only around seven of us on it – and it would help pass the time a bit. Other than that, I'd probably buy a loaf of bread and watch TV until they came back. Then on Sundays, we'd meet up in the pub.

In my second year of college, I came off my bike and dislocated my shoulder. I'd been out with my flatmates on Friday afternoon and said I'd race them back home – me on the bike and them lot in the car. It all started out OK until I came to a roundabout and went arse-over-tit as they say, over the handlebars, sprawled out on the road and in severe pain. As I sat in agony a man stopped to help and got me to hospital where they gave me a general anaesthetic and re-set it. After being away for ages, I got back to the house to find it empty. Everyone had just buggered off without even waiting or wondering where I was. I sat through such pain that weekend and felt so alone. I wasn't too chuffed on Sunday when they came back without any hint of concern.

Finishing at Barrow College just delayed the fact that I still had no career aspirations. Another pattern emerging here, eh? I know people who are in work now and still don't know what they want to do as a career, just going from job to job as a means to an end, so I know I'm not alone in that one. Like many of my friends at college, I applied to go into higher education and was offered a place on a degree course at Manchester Polytechnic to study Economics.

I moved with Mark into a place in Manchester but unfortunately we ended up falling out after a few weeks and I moved into Auntie Doreen's. I hate confrontation and falling out, so the opportunity to move in with her solved a problem for me. There had been a bit of tension with Mark over money for bills and keeping on top of the practicalities of living. He was always organised and I wasn't, so we got on each other's nerves a bit and it came to a head one day. He worked out on a Sunday how much we owed and, as I didn't have a cash card, I said I'd get the money out the bank the following day. When I'd got the money out and got back home, Mark was on me immediately asking if I had been to the bank. I thought it was a bit abrupt of him and told him that if the tension carried on I'd move out.

'Move out then,' was his reply. And I did.

I loved living with Auntie Doreen and she really looked after me well. Talk about being 'fed and watered' properly! She would cook my favourite meals day in, day out (sausage, liver and bacon casseroles were always top of the list) and made sandwiches for my lunch to take to poly. One day I told her that I liked haslet and subsequently had it in my sarnies every day for a month.

The dangerous thing was Auntie Doreen used to make the sandwiches for me the evening before, rather than rushing around in the morning. And then I would take them upstairs to 'pack' my bag. If the sandwiches ever did see the next day they would certainly be long gone by the time the bus had done a couple of stops. I just couldn't help myself. It was food and it was mine. On my way back early evening I would eat loads of crisps and sweets on the bus, even when I knew I'd be having a meal when I got to Auntie Doreen's. It didn't matter to me. I also used to visit the cafes in the city centre and would always sneak away from poly at any opportunity for cottage pie and chips.

I would still go to visit Mum and Dad quite often and liked to go when there was a home match so I could combine it with a trip to watch Barrow. I loved every aspect of going to the football; it was amazing and gave me such a buzz. It was round about this time that the love affair began to come to an end though, not because of the way they played – it was because it was starting to get difficult for me to stand up too long during the games. Despite this, every time I was at Mum's I would pop down to the pie shop for a bag of pies, eating a couple on the way back. Sometimes I would stand in the back street out of view to fill my face.

Not being able to stand for long was a worry. This was the first time I'd really felt the effect of being overweight. I know my size limited my athletic abilities anyway, but standing up is something everyone expects to be able to do. It was a horrible feeling, like in a Hollywood movie where snippets of dialogue segue into each other to shoehorn a point for the unintelligent audience. Suddenly I could see Mum bursting in on me cooking burgers in the caravan, I could hear the voices, the childhood parties, queuing up in the pie shops, see the looks from people in the street ...

Look at the size of him.

                    You're eating your own grave.
I've made your favourite.

                    You wouldn't be able to do that.
Charlie's is the one with the most on.

                    You'll be heavier than me soon.
I've saved some more for you.

                    The oldest student in the country.
Do you want some more, love?

                    When are you going to get a job?
Here's some pudding.

                    Don't you think you should go on a diet?
You fat bastard.

                    Why don't you ever play out with friends?
Look, he can hardly walk.

                    Those trousers look a bit tight for you.
You've put on weight.

                    Are you eating again?

I used to see Mark around college and he'd say hello
and I'd blank him. I was really hurt by the way he
went on, but if I was honest, it wasn't all one sided. I
was quite untidy and Mark is one of those perfection-
ists who have an immaculate house, and he's always
been like that. It was difficult for me because I'm not
the type who bears a grudge, so it was difficult to blank
someone I liked and wanted to be on speaking terms
again with.

But we cleared the air by talking for a long time
over too many cups of tea and, soon after, I moved back
in with him for my final year. It was getting a bit much
travelling from my auntie's every day, so it worked out
well for me. It was only years later that I found out
that Mark had been going through a really difficult
time personally when all this was kicking off and it

made me feel bad that he had had me adding to it all.

Feeling a bit optimistic, I decided I would lose some weight and Mark said he'd help me ... as if sitting my finals weren't stressful enough. My usual definition of 'cramming' is a bit different from the studious one and it was never easy just to sit at a desk and not pick at snacks in the process. In addition to this, Mark had taken a year out and we started to go out quite a lot (so much for the help!). I got a part-time job at the Top Rank bingo club in Newton Heath to help fund being able to live and, although it brought money in, it added to the chaos. As we know, losing weight needs discipline and a complete lifestyle change and, at that point, there was so much else going on. This is the excuse that's all too easy. How many times in the last week have you said you are too busy to do something? And it is usually the things that mean a lot: too busy to call or send a text message to someone, too busy to take time out to relax, too busy to read a book or to visit a friend. Although I actually did lose weight with the regime, it probably wasn't enough. I was still chubby, unattractive (in my eyes) and very shy. Losing the weight was an accomplishment that I just never saw. *You may have lost weight, but you're still fat.* It should have been a positive to keep me going. I'd always put my own spin on it and would always end up feeling bad rather than good.

When I finished my course I was disappointed to only get a 2:2. A Desmond is nothing to be sniffed at though. Mum and Dad and my Auntie Doreen came to the graduation and were as proud as punch. Wearing a mortar board and gown is enough to make anyone feel a bit silly. Once you see everyone on your way to the ceremony and meet up with people who are all dressed the same, your inhibitions leave and you feel an amazing sense of achievement. You are dressed like that for one big reason – you passed! I'd passed. I'd done it. I was the first Walduck with a degree and it *did* mean a lot to me. The other side to graduation is the job side: you have just been studying for three years to set you on the road to a lifetime's career. People from my course were talking about the job interviews they'd had since I last saw them, many had secured good jobs and told me of their plans and what they'd been up to.

'I have a job,' I said. 'I'm a bingo caller.'

Everyone it seemed, apart from me, was doing well for themselves and I was working for very low wages at the bingo club. I was getting left behind. They may have been friends for three years, but in the big, bad world, they were competition. Or not, as the case was. I don't know what they really made of my job, other than probably thinking I had no ambition, because with respect, it was a job I didn't need a degree in Economics for. From my point of view, it was a job I enjoyed doing and that counted for a lot. Was I so wrong not to be chasing a high-earning city job?

I didn't stay at Top Rank all that long and went to work at Mecca bingo club in Bury. The manager from Newton Heath moved jobs and asked if I'd go to work with him over there, so it was like being headhunted for the first time. This is when the weight started to pile back on, I would eat all the time and I got bigger and bigger again. I had a great time working there and made some wonderful friends though. I knew I was getting bigger, I knew I was eating too much, I knew exactly what was going on and what the problem was: I just did nothing about it. I was only interested in eating food, not trying to work it off. Exercise wasn't part of my lifestyle and I was reaching the point where even thinking about exercise was just ridiculous. I was a big lad, always had been, always would be. Pointless trying to change it.

Every Monday, Cynthia (the boss) and I would start a 'diet' and every Tuesday we'd have trifles from the cafe next door. It was a farce. I'd usually volunteer to get them just so I could eat a couple on the way back on the QT and then have the other in Cynthia's company; 'on the way back' literally being a few steps. I probably peaked at around thirty stone because of things like that. I was getting slower and less inclined to walk or go anywhere because of the effort it would take. This was taking me right into the danger zone. Just like the feeling I got about not being able to stand up for long, my mobility going downhill was something that I started to put up with rather than do something about. I did have spells of losing weight, which always went hand in hand with setbacks.

I once went on a sponsored weight loss and actually put weight on! How bad did I feel after that? As a forfeit, I had to call bingo dressed as a fairy. I didn't mind so much though; it made for a more entertaining evening. Every Friday night I would sing a song for the customers and dress up – I had always wanted to perform and it was a great excuse to do something I loved. It was like starring in panto every week.

Even though it was fun working there I would occasionally try and escape the bingo life and find something else. I'm not sure if it was out of curiosity, just to see if somewhere else wanted me, or if I actually did want another job ... or even the option of one. Maybe I just never felt completely happy anywhere I was. When I got knocked back, I would respond by knocking back the pies. To be fair, I never needed much of an excuse, but this was always my way of dealing with it. Self-harm, Walduck style. It was an extreme form of comfort eating, gorging out on all the fattiest foods known to humankind without a care for any of the associated long-term consequences. Overeating gave me the control in my life that I needed and calmed a situation down, bringing a sense of balance back. Food for me was like taking a razorblade and carving into my arm.

In 1995 I left Mecca and was offered a job at the Riva bingo hall in Belle Vue, a club I would work at for the next twelve years. It was sad to leave all my wonderful friends behind, especially Karen, Sue and Cynthia. I knew we'd always remember the laughs we had; I still think about it all even now.

No two days are ever the same working in a bingo hall and, over the years, I am proud to say I have met and made many great friends at all the places I've worked. I hope in some small way I made the customers' lives more fulfilled. That was something I always strived to do because the customers were everything to the industry. It was them who made it a community; a place to talk, to share conversation, to have a laugh and to just be part of something that meant, well ... it meant everything. A friendly greeting and a lovely smile makes all the difference, and knowing that the customers were happy always made me happy too. I was king of the double-edged compliment. It was all in the spirit of the night and we had a good laugh.

'You smell lovely tonight. What is it you're wearing, Domestos?'

'You've got the look of a Hollywood actress. Who is it I'm trying to think of ... Oh yes, Lassie.'

The old jokes are always the best and I loved the

banter we'd get going by having the punters heckle us. It was always about setting the joke up and everyone knowing there'd be a punchline coming – no matter how bad or old it was, the reception it received would still be good because people expected that kind of humour. It was never about making fun of someone or humiliating them because then I wouldn't have been doing my job properly; no one should feel uneasy on a night out.

This was why I wasn't in my graduate management scheme and plotting when I'd make my first million. Being part of that community made me feel good about myself. When I was calling bingo, I was in charge, I was cracking the jokes and I was making the night an enjoyable one. And that went a long way – people would approach me to talk about something I'd said, or say thanks, or carry on the laugh the next time they were back. That's what made it special. Then on the way home it would all be over and I'd be back to being the real me, back to an empty house and a fully stocked kitchen.

One misconception people always have with regards to bingo is that it's a game for elderly people – that is, until they experience the game for themselves and enjoy not only the chance of winning money, but also the social element. Bingo halls had a bit of a PR push in recent years to bring more people in. I mean, the money you can win is phenomenal. It's progressed so much over the years; you'd be amazed if you gave it a go. But that progression also looks like its downfall.

With everyone being on t'internet now and because of the smoking ban there are fewer and fewer people attending and more places closing down to make way for luxury apartments and shopping centres. And there are so many online incentives so that you don't need to leave the comfort of your own home to win just as much money. I'll stop now because I'm aware that I'm advertising online bingo when I'd much rather see more people getting out the house. The whole part of it in the first place was about creating an enjoyable social experience. Now it's like we're too busy for all that.

It never ceased to amaze me just looking at the mix of people and ages all under one roof. When there was a big win, there was never any jealousy; folk who played were always chuffed for those who won. No fighting, no arguing and swearing ... although some nights it would have been funny to see it all kick off with the oldies if some twenty year old won on their first go at playing.

I soon got to the point where it became difficult to find a uniform to fit me. I'd been living with this all my life, not necessarily feeling myself physically gaining the weight, but seeing all the reactions and feeling the strain of it on my being. My head was in the sand but the truth was that I was embarrassed by my size. My food consumption was growing all the time, much like the parallel of an addict's fix, needing more to satisfy all the time. There are not many people who are comfortable with telling people their clothing size for uniforms, even if they are what we call a 'normal' size. There'll always be someone slimmer waiting to give their measurements next. There's always the pressure to say a size smaller to save face a bit, but it just means your clothes won't be comfortable either. Nobody likes to admit that they can't fit into clothing.

I couldn't really get away with telling them I was a thirty-four-inch waist. Or even double that. The managers had to phone round to find suppliers of big clothes and I'd have to have my shirts specially made to measure because you couldn't buy my size anywhere, other than if you were planning a camping trip. See, I joke, but it was a harrowing thing for me to go through.

I remember being asked to take a coach load of customers on a holiday and I only had two shirts and one pair of trousers. I squeezed into the trousers and one of the shirts before going to meet all the other customers and staff from other clubs who'd gathered to go on the trip. The seats in the canteen had fixed middles and I knew I would not be able to fit. It was frustrating because in these situations it was designers and manufacturers of furniture that were alienating me, making a point that I was too fat to sit at one of their dining tables. I went and sat on an 'easy chair' that was anything but easy to sit in. As I sat, my shirt bulged open and the buttons were ready to pop under the strain. I looked down to see that a pen had leaked in my pocket, completely ruining the shirt and leaving a big blue patch. I was gutted. I was limited enough when I only had two shirts! Why did these things happen? Pens only leak in shirt pockets in comedies, not in real life.

I loved going on the holidays and would be very sad once they ended and it was time to go home. It was the same story – never wanting something good to end because it meant that I had to come back to reality. It was great to be there with everyone though; having a nice time and enjoying just socialising, away from it all. They were always a friendly bunch on those trips. I used to get upset when all the other staff members from the other clubs got dressed up and looked great whilst I could never get clothes to fit me. It was the only part I didn't enjoy about it.

It stands to reason that carrying so much excess weight around is not good for you and I was under no illusion.

It was difficult to move around, to 'just squeeze past' anyone or anything, to get upstairs, downstairs, to sit, stand, walk, lie down, get dressed, put shoes and socks on, have a bath or shower, get washed in general, get dried, go to the toilet. Anything. Anything you can think of was difficult. And it was all because of food.

The more weight I put on, the more stressed I became by it. I was in an impossible situation. I hated what I was and would sometimes take out my frustrations on my friends and colleagues by snapping at them. Not the best thing to do, really. I was angry with myself all the time and those close to me would be in the firing line. It felt worse because I knew I wasn't that kind of person. I don't go around shouting at people, but when I was consumed by this 'thing' I changed. I dare say that food had an impact on my mood too. I just know I was fed up, miserable ... all the negative connotations you can think of, I was them.

When walking round the club finally became too much of a chore, I would park myself on stage and would be set for the night. That's always a downside to having a job where you sit down for a living – any amount of food you eat is not getting burnt off through exercise. Then, in 1997, a chance came up for me to do something about it. I decided to retire from bingo calling and work on night security instead. I really thought it was a chance to lose weight, to be walking around constantly and start to change the way I lived.

It turned out that night security was just a way of being able to eat twenty-four hours a day instead. I hadn't been told this when I started, so imagine my delight when a delivery of cream cakes arrived first thing in the morning for the diner. The first time this happened it was like Santa had been! Or Satan.

Whichever. It was like a mirage. I had to rub my eyes – a massive tray full of gorgeous-looking cream cakes just sitting there, all of them calling out to me in such angelic voices: *We love you. Please take us in and eat us. No one will ever know.*

So ... I took them inside. And you know what? I *didn't* eat them. Honest, guv. I think it was the consequence of the embarrassment that stopped me. I took them down to the diner, although I did take a couple of them and leave the money. It was impossible to resist.

On my way home I used to go to one cafe and have a breakfast, then go to another and another if the need was still there. The venue change was because the guilt of sitting there amongst the same people and them seeing me eating plate after plate would have been too much. Not too long after, I got over that guilt. I didn't care what anyone thought, I didn't want the feeling of food being in my mouth to end. The taste of it, the feel of it was just so amazing. I'd only stop once I was completely satisfied, stuffed to the point of self-loathing. It wasn't guilt as such that stopped me; it was a feeling of disgust that I'd done it. After a night shift, I'd end up going home and sitting in front of TV and eating. And eating. I was no longer consuming the food, it was consuming me.

Inevitably, my health worsened through this and I may have gotten stuck into the routine if it wasn't for a girl at work called Anna telling me a story about a lad she knew who had died.

'He had to be lifted into the grave by a crane,' she said. 'He was so big when he died that the hospital reckoned his organs just collapsed.'

I could not believe what I was hearing. It was such a sad story. Was this going to happen to me? I didn't want to just keel over one day and then need a JCB to bury me. I decided right then – and told everyone – I was going to lose weight. That was it, I'd had enough. The signs were there and I didn't want to end up in that predicament. And that's what I did. It was the wakeup call I needed.

I turned my life round entirely. It felt good – I knew exactly what I had to do. And then, a couple of days later, I turned back to food. The moment had passed; the shock was over ... back to the same old routine, back to the rut I didn't want to be stuck in. It was pretty pathetic, really. The worst part was that I always had these eureka moments when I'd announce to everyone that I, Charles Ambrose Walduck, was going to transform himself. Maybe the first time someone may have thought I meant it ... not after I'd said it ten times though. I don't blame them for having no faith in me. It must have been sad for them to see the enthusiasm on my face, saying this time it was different, and them knowing that at best I'd resist a cream cake or pie for a couple of hours.

Working overnight was clearly bad for me, so I decided to rejoin the land of the living on the daytime shift and started to feel better immediately. That was, until I was sat calling the numbers one day and felt my heart miss a beat. I didn't think too much of it and just carried on. A couple of minutes later I felt it again. *Oh my God*, I thought. *I am having a heart attack.* It got worse over the next couple of weeks. Then one Monday night I sat down in the office at work and knew something was wrong. My heart was beating irregularly all the time and I just sat there sobbing, panicking, helplessly. An ambulance was called and I was taken to hospital for an ECG.

'Your heart is fine, Mr Walduck,' the doctor told me. 'But you need to lose some of this weight.'

I was so delighted to be given the all clear. I knew after such a scare that I'd make a conscious effort – 'doctor's orders' and all that. After Anna's story and then this, I really did have to give myself a shake and get into shape. I caught the bus home, went to the shop en route and, knowing I'd be starting the diet tomorrow, bought myself a couple of pork pies, just to see me through. A couple more couldn't do any harm, eh?

At work the next day I was sat in my usual spot on stage calling bingo and I began having palpitations again. I left work in a panic and went to the doctor immediately. He told me he would put me on a heart monitor for twenty-four hours and do some blood tests. It seemed the irregular heartbeat was being caused by stress and anxiety. I knew I was stressed, and being told that by a doctor just stressed me out even more.

I'd moved to my present address in Failsworth, Manchester, not long before the palpitations, so I put a lot of the stress down to moving house. A house move can be a bit stressful, but I wouldn't have said it was that bad; certainly not bad enough to affect my heart. Without making any of the changes I kept promising, without exercising, dieting or making any real attempt at even small changes, my health was bound to get worse. At this point I'd stopped functioning as a human being in so many ways and it was like my body was starting to close down on me because I was abusing it so much.

It wasn't just because of not being able to stand that I'd stopped going to the football. There was a chronicle of events that led the way, all of them not nice to recall. It had been increasingly difficult to squeeze through the turnstile and I no longer wanted to suffer the indignity of trying to. It'll be difficult for many to comprehend this. Try to imagine the anguish building up when you are in a queue ... and then the inevitable: the looks from the stewards as they mentally prepare for the struggle, the shame as those in the queue nudge their friends and point, waiting for the struggler to get through, the ultimate embarrassment of either getting stuck or not coming close to fitting. Then the queue would be held up and grow impatient because I was blocking the turnstile. Simply being told not to bother trying hurt just as much. It was always a home loss to Walduck as he'd end up going for an early bath (so to speak – don't get me started on actually trying to fit into the bath).

There was a bloke I knew who worked for St John's Ambulance at Stockport Football Club. He was also a big lad and any time he was near or on the pitch he'd get shouted at too. The thing is with him, he had the confidence to let it go over his head and revel in the chanting and not let it get to him. He'd take his top off in bars and would dance around to the chanting too – completely mad as a hatter but completely happy in his skin. Or that's the impression he gave. It was maybe a defence mechanism to deflect and diffuse the ridicule. The fact is that people still gave him a hard time whether he could take it or not and it still wasn't fair. So what, you have to join in with the bullies and laugh at yourself, then cry behind closed doors?

It wasn't exclusive to just football fans though, anyone can be heartless if they put their tiny mind to it. I'd regularly get abused in the street – people driving past, beeping their car horn and shouting something derogatory before speeding off. Walking past any group of people, it was a certainty that someone within it would shout something at me.

But I don't just blame the narrow minded and ill

informed. People ridicule others for all sorts of reasons: to feel better about themselves, to cover up their own insecurities, because they have no manners, were brought up that way, or just to have a laugh at others' expense.

Then we have the influence the media has over public opinion. Celeb mags aren't as bad as they once were because they do have a balanced view now – showing celebs who have put on weight as well as the ones who have lost too much. There is more of a social conscience these days and their main view is that it isn't good to be too fat or too thin. But pick up any tabloid newspaper and the way they label fat people is rarely balanced – rolly-polly, lardy, lard arse, tubby – whatever description they use, it's picking fault at someone because of their weight. It usually is targeting someone 'bad', but all this does is fuel negativity towards fat people.

It also gets me quite angry when I see celebrities in magazines after they've just lost a couple of stones, telling us how great they feel having sorted themselves out once and for all. Then they'll be back a few months later when they've put it on again, and again when they've lost it. It's always the same couple of stones, and usually the same celebrities. What's the point, other than to sell more magazines?

It's through celeb culture and sites such as Pop Bitch that we now have a much better understanding of how the media works. The 'celeb frolicking on the beach' shot is rarely not set up in advance and the stars are working with the photographers or magazines that they usually claim to hate. But, as consumers of pop culture, we lap all this up. We love reading about

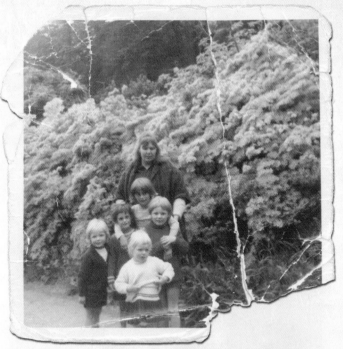

Mum, Jackie and Steven and a couple of cousins (I'm in blue).

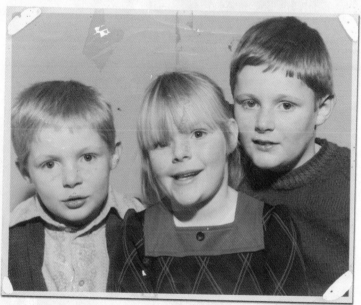

Steven, Jackie and me in one of those great school photos.

Me on the beach in Torquay. Russell (cousin), Steven, Philip (cousin) and me in the Wombles shirt ... it would probably be retro cool to wear that now, but it definitely wasn't in the 1970s!

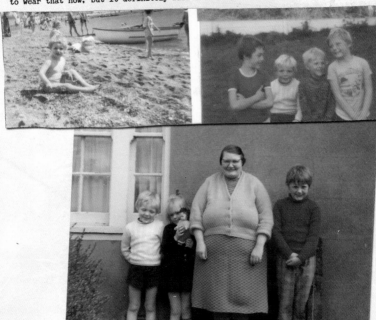

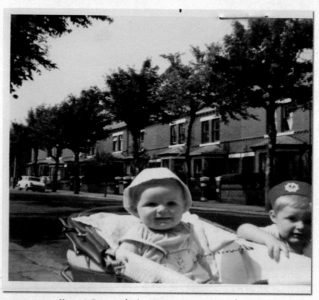

Steven, Jackie, Auntie Margaret and me
(no, I'm not off to a fancy dress party as Rupert the Bear).

Me and Steven (he's the one in the pram).

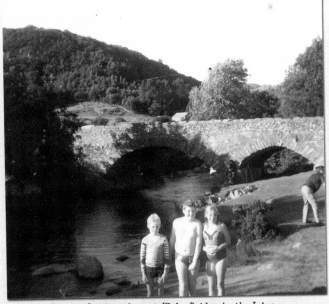
Steven, Jackie and me at Ulpha Bridge in the Lakes.

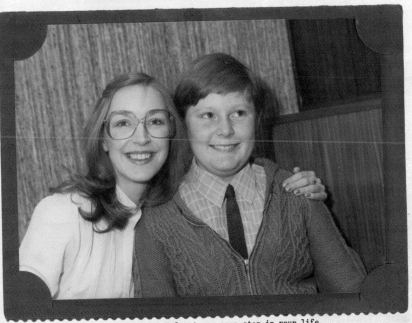
You have to meet at least one soap star in your life.
Here's me with Deirdre (Anne Kirkbride) from *Corrie*.

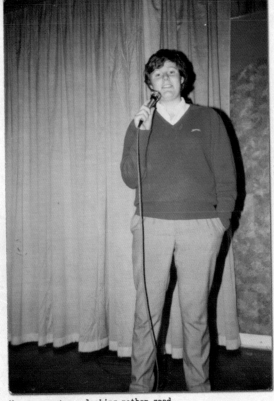

Me at seventeen, looking rather good.
I was always comfortable being behind a microphone.

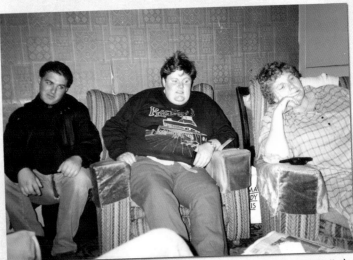

About a year later and not looking too good (my cousin Russell, me and Mum).

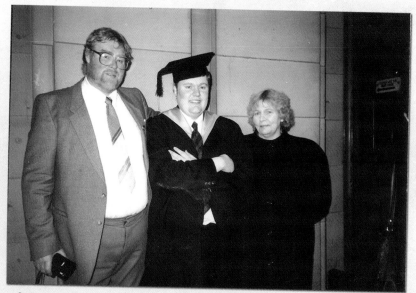

Dad, me and Mum at my graduation in 1991 ... another time when I had managed to lose some weight with the help of Mark. It wasn't long before I was eating again.

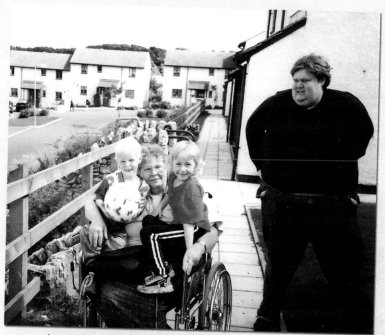

Around 1997, squeezed into those jeans and caught off guard (Mum with nephew Josh and niece Jade).

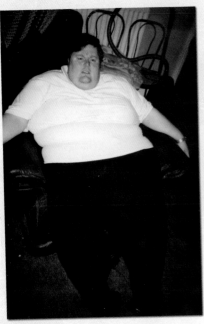

Relaxing in the chair in 2002.

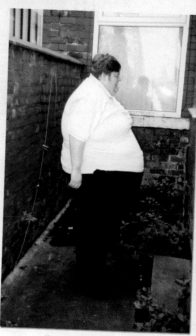

Not as relaxed outside.

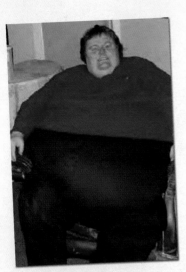

December 2003.
Smiling and yet desperately unhappy.

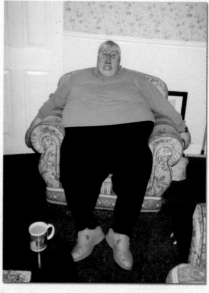

We all dyed our hair for the 2002 World Cup.
I thought I looked great, but photos never lie.

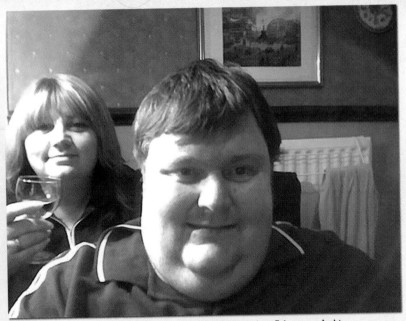

With Lucy, one of my best mates. Without her I have no doubt
I would not be here to tell my story.

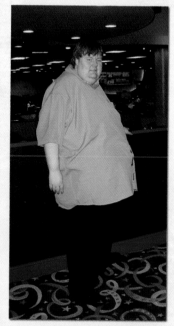

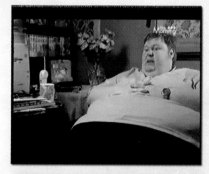

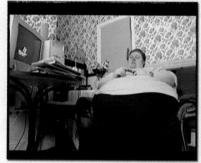

At the bingo and looking smart.
I'd lost around ten stones at this point.

From my story broadcast on *This Morning*.

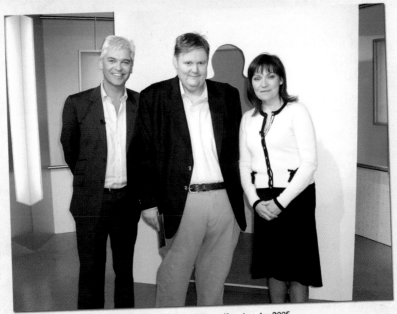

Phillip and Lorraine on *This Morning* in 2005
(I'd lost twenty-one stones at this point).

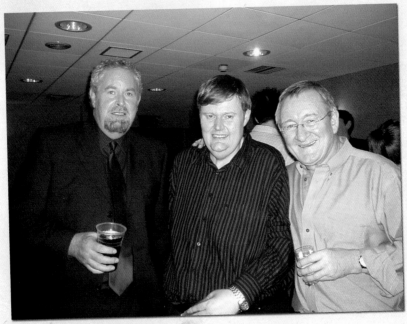

Jerry Kelly (left), me and Dr Chris on *The Jerry Kelly Show*.

who's been at the pies every week and we love to see the photos of it as evidence.

Then there are those other celebs – the ones who have had surgery – that have had their fair share of good and bad publicity. Once I'd lost my weight and become known as an 'ambassador for the obese', I'd get asked my opinion on the surgery debate. I'm always reluctant to criticise anyone, having faced it all my life.

Some people may genuinely find it impossible to train their mind to make them want to stop eating or may not have the motivation to do exercise. If surgery is what'll work for you, then it's fine. I'd maintain that I'm living proof that anyone can lose weight the non-surgical way, though.

What I don't like is when someone who's had surgery suddenly becomes the voice of the fatties. I don't think you can be if you haven't lost weight the non-surgery way. Having a band fitted means that you cannot physically eat any more than the band allows, so you cannot overeat. It's impossible. Can you speak for the obese and about the problems they face from that position? I don't think so.

I didn't know it then, but I'd soon be at a point in my life where I'd have to make changes or die. It was that simple. You can't carry on taking that kind of physical abuse for too long, and I was nearing the end. If you think about how alcoholics are told that their next drink could be their last, it was the same with me. Each pie, each greasy, stodgy piece of food I gorged on could have been my last. When you are aware of the risks and you still carry on, you know you're on borrowed time.

I've always had that New Year depression that people often moan about. Mine is a real depression though, rather than an off-the-cuff comment by the water cooler on a dark January morning. The year 2003 began pretty much the same for me: the thought of the coming months, the dull days, dark nights, the miserable weather, isolation, desolation and the constant need to comfort eat filled me with a sense of impending dread. When I was on a real low, there was nothing that could bring me round.

By February, I was the heaviest I had been in my entire life. I was just under fifty stone in weight and my future, if there was one, was bleak. At the start of each day I would regularly telephone the local cafe and order two or even three full breakfasts to be delivered. I had no qualms about leaving the front door open as I was completely happy for the delivery service to bring my food straight through to the living room. Let's face it – by the time I'd heaved myself off and out of the chair, up, through the house and opened the door, the delivery guy would have either given up or the food would have been cold. It was easier and it meant I got my food quicker. At the back of my mind, I was beginning to think about just staying in bed and having it delivered as a breakfast in bed. It would have made life even easier for me. The temptation was very strong, but luckily something held me back and thank goodness it did. Perhaps it was the thought of the shame to my family and friends and knowing that if I started doing that it would have signalled the end. I have no doubt that I'd have died in my bedroom from eating and eating. Having food delivered started to feel like some seedy drug deal. Like I was an incapable junkie who needed his fix brought to him. They'd bring the food in, I'd pretend there were other people in the house that the food was also for, and it became such a farce. We all knew there was no one else in the house; we all knew I had no kids or friends. And to turn it into even more of a freak show, the bloke who delivered the food actually brought his family round to look at me. That was a real low because they didn't even pretend to hide why they were there. It was to gawp.

It's always expected that I have no feelings, being this size – but to have people come round and gawp when you are at your lowest is disgusting. I was helpless, couldn't do anything about it, couldn't react ... I just wanted my fix.

A Typical Day in the Life of an Overeater

At my heaviest, I'd get up at around ten in the morning. It was never the best sleep in the world because there was always discomfort and restlessness. Sometimes I'd wake up at a daft time like five in the morning and go downstairs to my chair to sleep. I had two walking sticks to use to get out of bed. Pushing myself up could sometimes take a good while – ten minutes, twenty, an hour. It all depended on how my mood and energy was first thing. It was like having a workout as soon as waking up. I would always go to the toilet first thing because if I went downstairs first I always had to think about my energy reserves and whether I could make another trip. As bad as it is to admit, I couldn't wipe my arse properly. This is another downside to being so big. I had to lay a towel on my bed and sit, roll and manoeuvre myself and do the best I could. To get washed, I couldn't get in the bath and didn't have a shower, so this was another laborious task. I used to get through more talc than Pablo Escobar.

All the things you take for granted become the impossible when you reach that size, and take a dozen times longer to do. It was just something I learnt to cope with over the years – once you realise you can't do something, you have to look at ways around it and improvise when you need to. I got in touch with Social Services to get some help with having a shower installed and they agreed to pay a hundred pounds towards the installation. The whole cost was a couple of thousand anyway, so didn't go ahead with it. I used to get sores under my stomach and they'd cause me a lot of discomfort. My belly hung right down and I'd have to move it out the way to wash and to go to the toilet. And the sores used to smell bad too – like rotting, dying skin – and I had a big sponge to wash as best I could, then back to the bed to roll around in more talc before getting dressed.

I had only two jumpers, red for at home and blue for at work. Lucy had cut an old Gala Bingo polo shirt up to get the logo and then stitched it on to my sweatshirt. And I had two pairs of jogging bottoms with an eighty-two-inch waist, bought from a company online and both of which had seen better days. The drawstring snapped in them a long time ago, giving me an extra couple of inches. I didn't wear any socks because I couldn't physically put them on and I'd wear slip-on shoes because I could no longer tie laces either. My feet used to swell up a lot and some days it would take twenty minutes just to get them on. I always got them a size too big. At least it meant I didn't have to deliberate over what to wear every morning: red or blue on top, same old jogging bottoms, same old shoes. Easy, yet far from ideal.

I'd phone a taxi as I prepared to put my shoes on and it would usually arrive just as I was ready to go.

The taxi company knew exactly who it was and where I'd be going just by me saying, 'Hi, it's the big fella.'

I'd always carry a plastic bag around with a few essentials in. One of these was a tea towel that I'd put down on the passenger seat of the taxi. They'd always put the seat as far back as it would go and recline it to a virtual horizontal position so I could fit. Every time I got the towel out, I'd make an excuse up. I'd usually say it was because I'd just put my pants on from the wash and they weren't completely dry. I don't know if they ever had their own theory. The real reason behind using the towel was because I was terrified that I'd missed something when I was trying to clean myself and would be mortified if I left anything behind on the seat.

Once at work, I'd walk over to the reception desk and lean on it for a bit to catch my breath and recompose after around a minute's worth of walking. If my friend Billy was at work, I'd usually sit on the settee at reception for a bit of a chat and then he'd help me get up. I'd take another rest at the counter where they used to sell the bingo books and make my way down to the stage after that. This usually took around twenty minutes. Even the oldies could do it quicker. And at this point, nothing was about food. I'd not have eaten anything since waking up and might have a cup of tea when I was on stage. Sometimes, if I was that hungry, someone would bring me a fishcake down from the diner, having carried it in their pocket. It was pretty unhygienic, but what the hell. I wasn't going to refuse a fishcake just because it had a bit of pocket fluff stuck to it.

I'd work from eleven in the morning until my tea break at around three o'clock. The food that was served in the bingo hall, or any I've worked at or been in for that matter, has never been for the health conscious. I mean, the 'healthy option' generally meant a bit of salad in your burger.

Tea breaks meant making my way back to reception and sitting on the settee for two and a half hours. It was pointless and too expensive to go home for this amount of time. I'd usually sit with Beryl and she'd bring food in for us and I'd bring a few things in too. If anyone so much as moved, I'd always ask them to get me something, always wanting to know what shop they were going to. 'Can you just get me ...'

After my break, I'd sit with Sue at reception to meet and greet before being on stage at half past seven to call the numbers again. I'd also have the odd nap during breaks because of my disturbed and restless nightly sleep pattern. I bet I looked a right state, nodding off in my chair until being woken up by the regulars to get back to work.

At the end of a shift, there'd usually be food left over from the kitchen diner – plates of burgers and fish-cakes. They'd tell me to help myself as it would just be thrown out otherwise, so I'd be straight in and would eat as much as I could before bagging the rest for when I got home. I don't know if they were having a bit of a laugh at my expense, seeing my eyes light up and chuckling about me taking the leftovers home, or if it was out of kindness. It mustn't have bothered me that much because I still took them. I had the last laugh when I made off with my plunder.

On my way back home I'd ask the taxi driver to stop off at the garage so I could stock up on some food. Garages aren't really known for their healthy options, so the kind of stuff I'd get would always be pasties, pies, crisps, chocolate – all convenience rubbish to satisfy that night's craving. As time wore on, I got too big to get out of the taxi at the garage, and the taxi drivers ended up going in for me instead. They must have cringed at drawing the short straw on a night. And then, rather than making a pit stop, it became easier for the taxi driver to order a takeaway and swing by to pick it up. It was certainly easier for me and the food intake kept progressing all the time. Sometimes I'd be falling asleep in front of the TV, still eating my supper, but would rarely give up.

That was what my routine consisted of and my days off were on Wednesday, Thursday and Saturday. That was when the real eating took place.

The cafe on the corner of the street, as you now know, was great for fry-ups. I'd order a couple of breakfasts, a burger, a pie and some cakes over the phone and they'd deliver it straight to the door. I'd get them to chuck a knife and fork in because I never had the energy to go to the kitchen. It would be fifteen quid for that little lot and sometimes I'd ask them to stick one or two cups of tea in there as well. This was the place where I'd pretend I was ordering for me and 'my guest'.

I'd get my shopping delivered from one of the supermarkets online. I'll not mention them by name in case they send me free food as a thank you. Online shopping is brilliant in some respects and bad in others. For starters, it meant that I was even less likely to leave the house than before and meant I had an excuse to stay in because I couldn't miss the delivery. And once it arrived, more often than not, I used to sit and eat most of it, if not all, depending if all of it was instant gratification or had to be cooked. It was very likely that most of it wouldn't make it to the cupboard, fridge or freezer. If there was a place online where they brought you the food, cooked it and served you it, you can bet your life I'd have been on it.

I'd sit in on a night, lonely and miserable. I've always been single – never had a partner to share my life with and have always wanted to know what it's like to be in love with someone and in a relationship. I knew I'd never go anywhere where I'd be likely to meet someone and always felt I was missing something in my life. And of course, there I was every night filling that void with food. I'd just eat and eat until it hurt. There was no pleasure in it. At my low points, I'd crumple any leftovers up, smother it with ketchup or the dregs from a cup of tea so it would be destroyed and disgusting, and throw it in the bin. This was so I wouldn't be tempted to try to eat it, but sure enough, there were times when I retrieved and ate it.

Other than a routine of work, there was nothing. When I was off work, I would get up, order food and just sit. And sit. Then, when I began to feel more depressed because of how I looked and felt, I'd take time off work and just sit. Eating and sleeping was all I had in times like this. When I got to the point of hardly being able to move, then this was another reason for staying off work and locking myself away. My days were spent battling with my inner turmoil and all of these battles were lost. The forfeit was always to overeat. At least when I was at work there were fewer opportunities, although I'd always make up for it whenever I could.

I had huge, horrible, weeping ulcers on my legs that wouldn't heal up. I was in constant agony and getting up on a morning was such a miserable start to the day. I used to have a metal-framed bed that had been quite sturdy until one night it collapsed under my weight. It had been a bit of a rude awakening, but there was very little I could do about it at stupid o'clock in the morning so it was a problem that I just slept on, pardon the pun. After a while, I got someone to take the bed frame away, leaving me with just the mattress on the floor. And that was how I slept from then on, making it a thousand times harder to get out of on a morning. Sometimes it could take anywhere up to two hours, with having to manoeuvre myself and roll to the edge of the mattress and struggle to get to a sitting position. I'd be knackered doing this. I often imagined that one day I might not be able to do it; that I'd die there on my mattress having not been able to move, not having had the energy to quite make it.

The walking sticks I mentioned earlier were to help heave myself up and it became a bit more manageable that way. I got them after falling over in the bathroom one day and not being able to get back up. Stuck for two hours, I had to crawl my way out and was scared I was going to die there. The desperation of being alone in that situation is difficult to recall. The energy it took to crawl, pulling myself along on my own floor, having to keep stopping, having to muster up more energy all the time, fearing that if I gave up I'd be dead. I would have been one of those sad stories like Anna had told me, a newspaper article or an embarrassing addition to the local news. This was another time where I should have done something about it.

The 'should haves' were growing all the time and my life turned into a desperate mess, a tale of how not to live, a textbook-style 'I told you so.' And all the time, there was a catalogue of missed opportunities to lose weight. All I had to do was realise I was killing myself and do something about it, really. Until then I was quite blissfully ignorant about my 'condition'. Yes, I knew I wasn't in the peak of my physical prime, but when your legs are covered in sores, it is time to begin to accept some responsibility and try to seek help.

In all honesty, because of my obesity, I'd never even known a 'physical prime' in my life. My legs continued to get worse and change colour and, as I had nothing better to do, one day I got out my medical dictionary. A few minutes later and Dr Walduck had the full diagnosis: blocked arteries, not enough blood getting through my legs to my feet, no pulse in my feet ... I was going to lose my legs. I managed to convince myself of that. This only led to further panic because I refused to go to see a real doctor and seek help, knowing that I'd be told the inevitable.

Lucy, one of my dear and closest friends, came round to my house each day without fail, bringing with her antiseptic lotions and creams, purchased from the chemist or acquired from friends and family. She would tenderly bathe and dress my disgusting legs to help relieve the pain and misery. They say true friends are hard to find and Lucy is quite simply one of the best. I will never forget all she has done for me.

I really felt like she was saving my life. It must have been difficult for her, and for her to keep a brave face and try to lift my spirits. I even bought some healthy food in a desperate bid to lose weight and save my legs, and then two days in I thought, *What the hell. I don't use my legs anyway so what's the point in trying to save them?*

One evening I phoned my mum. I guess I was at my lowest ebb and in the depths of depression because I never gave any thought to her feelings as I poured out my heart and complained about everything that was bad in my life. I told her that I was so sick of living in this body, so sick of being me that I just wanted to end it all. I couldn't see a way out. How could I lose it all if I couldn't even move? Just sit there and eat salads all day until I shrunk?

It must have been horrific, being told all that by your son. I began with my weight, then my ill-health, the state of my finances and the atrocious state of the house, which because of my lack of mobility had been left to go to rack and ruin.

That night was probably the longest of my life. I watched the seconds and minutes slowly tick by, riddled with pain, every tortuous movement inducing more tears of anguish and remorse. What a pitiful creature I was; what a self-deprecating slob I had become. I hated myself and everything I was. I looked around and was disgusted that I'd ended up this way: a grown man who'd eaten so much all his life that he couldn't move, couldn't even get out of a seat to tidy his own mess up, couldn't even have a proper wash because he was too fat to have a bath or shower and couldn't even wipe his own arse properly if he went to the toilet. I was so ashamed of myself.

A few minutes later, Mum phoned back and said she was on her way over to see me. It was such a relief to know that Mum would help. She talked to me and comforted me; she cleaned my house from top to bottom. She herself had mobility issues, but that didn't bother her one bit. She never complained; she came in and got on with the job. My throat was dry, my fists were clenched and I failed to fight the tears back while I sat watching, helplessly. It pains me to recall the vision, and this may help you understand how much mental torture I endured: Mum had to get on her hands and knees to do all the housework, crawling around in all my mess to clean up after me.

Mum had a fall in the street years earlier and was never quite the same. She used to always go to town on a Friday, and when we'd grown up a bit and didn't go any more she continued going on her own. She'd slipped on a strawberry in Barrow market. After the fall, she could never walk without getting the sensation that she was falling and became scared of walking. It was like severe vertigo. We used to say it was in her head, meaning that she just thought she was going to fall but wasn't actually in danger, but Mum took it that we meant she was making it up. It must have been horrible for her. She can't really walk at all. She'd hold Dad's hand for a bit, then she used to hold on to other people. At my graduation in 1991 she used a walking stick, which she did for a time until Dad got her a wheelchair; typically, one that was too big to fit through doorframes in houses.

Mum also motivated me into having the guttering at the front of the house repaired. Every time there was rain, it would pour down the walls in the living room. My gas boiler was broken at this time too – it had a big British Gas sticker on it saying 'Do not use' so I was without central heating and hot water and the house became damp and smelled because of it. She stayed with me all that week and, when Dad came to pick her up, he brought me a pair of slippers. I was more or less bedridden at this point and he came up to see me and put the slippers on my feet. He never used to lecture me about losing weight. He'd always say 'Do the necessary and look after yourself' and I'd always say 'I will, I will' and never did. It must have been difficult for him all the other times, but I'm sure that this one had been the worst. It was like he was coming to see me on my death bed. An animal suffering like this would have been put to sleep long before.

Mum got in touch with Social Services too and arranged for a cleaner to come around once a week to help out. This also added to the shame: having to alert the council to the fact that I was in no fit state to look after myself. She also made me go to the doctor, where I was given anti-depressants and felt I'd taken my first step on the road to recovery. Mum's only reward for all her hard work was the promise from me that I would try to lose weight. And after putting my mind to it, I did lose weight. And after finally overcoming my fear of the doctor, I started to feel much better. I was determined this time. I was going to turn it all round and really make a go of getting my act together. The start was made, I was feeling good and I stuck to a plan.

And then I destroyed it all again. I don't know what made me feel the worst, letting Mum and Dad down again or letting myself down again. I certainly couldn't have felt any worse if I'd tried. When the weight was put back on, when the promises became empty, when I reverted back to living like a slob with no self-respect, all that misery and depression came back a thousand times worse. I was convinced this time that there really wasn't anything I could do. I'd tried so many times and made so many promises. No one would believe me anymore. Why would they? And why would they even bother to help me? I just said anything anyone wanted to hear to their face while in private had my finger hovering over the self-destruct button.

And speaking of a thousand times worse, that gives me a perfect link to what happened in August that year. It was a spate of bad luck that I didn't think was ever going to end. The first straw was a visit from my sister, Jackie. As a result of a recent split with her boyfriend, she decided to come and stay with me for a short break. I like my own space, but when a family member is in need, you do what you can, and although I love my sister dearly it wasn't long until we were bickering. This led to a few nasty arguments and harsh words, none of which need to be repeated, and it's safe to say we both gave as good as we got.

At the time, Jackie was drinking rather more than she should have been and this added to the tension in the house. She was obviously upset about the breakup and I think I became the focus of her attention. From day one she took control – I think she thought she could be my saviour. I, on the other hand, wanted nothing more than to be left alone in peace and quiet. I couldn't be bothered with it all, especially when we both knew she was there for a short period of time and I would have been a part-time project to get left behind when she went back home.

One evening I took her along with me to work, hoping she'd enjoy a few games of bingo and forget about her problems for a bit. They'd still be there the next day, so a night off from all that wouldn't hurt. Unfortunately, I've never owned a crystal ball. I'd never had the need for one until after that night. Even more unfortunately, I exchanged some rather harsh words with a work colleague over something quite trivial, but nevertheless the argument was overheard by Jackie. It was something that needn't have happened; you know how these things escalate.

After my shift was over, I decided to take Jackie to the local pub where I'd heard that many of my work colleagues would congregate to round off the evening. Of course, I chose the wrong evening and the pub was completely empty. If I'd bothered to go out with them instead of being in a rush to get home and eat, I'd probably have known this was not a night they'd be there. We stayed anyway and Jackie had a bit more to drink and, whether it was the result of too much alcohol or not, Jackie was soon quite animated and decided to give me some home truths.

In her opinion, I was a complete waste of space with no friends to speak off. She went on to say that it was evident that I was disliked by work colleagues too. Her contempt on that evening was all too clear and I was deeply upset. They say alcohol allows you to say what you really want. Well, I certainly found out firsthand that night!

Completely demoralised, I once again turned to my friend Lucy. She was quick to reassure and promptly invited me, Jackie one of Jackie's friends to her house for a meal the following evening to see if we could rebuild a few bridges. This could have gone either way: potential for Jackie and me to make up or a venue for round three. And it was also the perfect opportunity to wear my new white shirt that I was dead chuffed with. As I pulled the delicate material over my body, it clung to me like a second skin. I started to feel really self-conscious about it. Despite this, when I looked in the mirror, I remember thinking how smart I looked. You can't beat the buzz of something new to wear and I felt good for a change. I've since looked back on photographs taken that evening and I cannot believe how deluded I was. I looked horrendous.

Lucy, as always, proved to be the perfect host. The food was superb, the drinks were flowing and once again Jackie soon got tired and emotional. And then she got to the point where it was quite embarrassing. It's never nice when you take someone to a friend's house and they get hammered. I knew Lucy didn't blame me, but I did feel responsible for it. This took the evening from bad to worse and eventually the taxi arrived to take me, Jackie and her friend home. I was so relieved to get out of that situation.

As Jackie got louder and louder, the taxi driver became really annoyed, to the point where he couldn't take any more and ordered us out of the cab. You know you're bad when someone who is used to driving drunks around actually throws you out his car! And it makes it difficult to get another cab to pick you up. How good was this for my stress levels? We were dumped unceremoniously outside a petrol station a good distance from home and Jackie then decided she needed the toilet. As there wasn't one around, she made do with the forecourt (who said the Walducks aren't classy?). There are not many things more annoying than trying to keep a drunk in order ... trying to keep two in order beats it hands down though. Jackie and her mate were rolling around all over the place, shouting and laughing, and it was turning into a nightmare.

My legs were really aching and I longed to be home and safe in bed. The night was dragging on forever and I thought I was never going to get home, but we eventually managed to secure another taxi. To my complete humiliation, it took both Jackie and her friend to ungraciously pull and tug and drag me out of it and inside the house.

I vowed there would never be a repeat performance of such a disastrous evening. It was a great relief when Jackie reconciled her differences with her boyfriend, packed her bags and left for home. She's my sister, I love her, but there's no way we could both exist in the same house without us driving each other mad! I'm sure she'd agree. I still haven't got round to getting the crystal ball either.

Without wanting it to start sounding like my catch-phrase, things then went from bad to worse. If ever there was a time for needing a crystal ball, this would have been it. August 2003, and roughly a week before my thirty-fifth birthday, it was my turn to be on reception at the club. This meant I'd be taking tele-phone calls and issuing temporary membership cards. It was a Tuesday night. Beryl would always make something for us to eat on Tuesdays and we'd sit and have our break together. Any day ending in a 'y' was food day. It's funny how you build up routines and the slightest thing can cause a huge change. Our breaks would always consist of sandwiches and I'd usually have a pork pie and crisps along with it. I'd then make the trip from the settee (which I used to more or less fill) over to my chair in reception to work with Sue. Not the most thrilling routine in the world, I'll give you that, but a routine all the same.

My chair only had one arm as the other had come off, but it was comfortable and nobody else would ever sit on it because it was my chair. I later discovered the real reason: it was because it smelt so bad from me sitting on it. Working with Sue always entailed having a right good laugh, talking, singing songs, messing around making fun of the customers. We'd make fun of them in a friendly way, and usually with them, so they'd join in – never anything bad behind their backs. And this night in particular, it seemed that *everyone* was in, so there were plenty of people stopping by for a chat. It was sometimes easy to leave your troubles outside and lose yourself in the fun of the evening and this night was one of them.

At around 7.20pm I was getting ready to make the short but difficult journey from reception to my chair up on the stage. I was still smiling as I began to heave myself up, then I glanced over to the main doors to see three men wearing balaclavas burst into the club and straight toward me. They had axes and bricks with them and looked very dangerous as they strode toward me purposefully. I stood off my chair as they approached – I have no idea what was going through my mind – and they demanded money. I was gripped by fear, cemented to the spot. The foyer was completely empty apart from us and there was no way of alerting anyone. I had absolutely no idea what to do. I couldn't run, hide or fight them. I couldn't give them money because there wasn't any.

I hope you never find yourself in this situation. Believe me, having three masked blokes with brandished weapons demanding money from you is the most frightening experience. I was numb. It wasn't a clichéd 'slow motion' situation either, just so surreal and terrifying. I said something to the effect that I didn't have any money there and one of them smashed me hard in the face. It was so quick, I didn't know if it was a punch or I was struck with an axe handle. I fell to the floor and I knew I wouldn't be able to get up. There I lay, helpless, waiting for the inevitable kicking. A brief silence followed before I heard more commotion and Sue shout 'They've hit Charlie!' The would-be robbers threw the brick in my direction and made off, empty-handed.

I was left really shaken that night. It's the last thing you expect to happen and it made me feel really vulnerable in a place where I used to feel safe and secure. I was convinced they were going to come back and hurt me. I mean, I was the one who foiled their plans, and revenge would be quite easy as they knew where I worked and what I looked like. All that was going through my mind was *Why me? Why me?* It was almost like they'd waited until I was alone, like I was targeted. It sounds a bit selfish, but it was typical that I was the only one for it to happen to, the only one to get punched.

The next day I had a massive bruise practically covering my face. To deflect the incident and to help me cope, I made jokes about it at work. The truth was it took all the courage I could find just to walk back into the club. I don't mind admitting I was still terrified. I was on the stage calling the numbers by 7.30pm and joked to the customers that I would have given the men the money if the customers hadn't kept winning it all. When the interval came I managed to make my way to the toilet and, once inside, I locked myself in the cubicle and broke down in tears. It was a delayed reaction to extreme trauma. I'd never felt so desperate, alone and stripped of my dignity. I had one of the worst panic attacks I'd known and phoned Mum.

I was terrified those men would find out where I lived and come round to finish me off. For all I knew they were in the audience, listening to me sneering at them, and had followed me to the toilets. I felt useless and wanted to die. I went home and sat with tears rolling down my face, thinking about my life, wiping at the tears with one hand and holding a packet of crisps with the other. I read on the Teletext service about the robbery and there was no mention of me being injured. It was if I never mattered. You read about robberies and they always say if someone was injured but not this time; even crime reporters overlooked me. The police were due to come back the next day and take pictures of my injury, but they never did. Why would anything that happened to me matter to anyone? Who was really bothered that I was injured? Who'd really have cared if they'd come after me and smashed my skull in with their axes? I remember the police asking me on the night how old I was and I told them it would be my birthday next week. I think that made it worse because birthdays always conjured up such happy thoughts for me, yet here I was in the depths of despair with my next one just around the corner.

I still think about it all now. I suppose some people would say that this would be another spur to lose weight, but in actual fact it almost tipped me over the edge. It made me question myself and my existence even more than usual. Would things have turned out differently if I had not been so grossly overweight? Perhaps I could have been a hero instead of a snivelling overweight wreck. I replay the scene over and over in my head and reflect how quickly my life could have ended that evening.

The third and final incident also happened on a Tuesday night a couple of weeks later.

As usual I was sat on my chair on the stage, ready to call the evening session at good old Gala. Behind the microphone, I was comfortable and I was in control. I always liked being in that position because I had power. People listened to me. Customers laughed and joked with me, but above all else, and I guess what meant the most, was that, up there on my throne, the customers respected me. I don't mean I loved the power in the sense that I'm some sort of tyrant ... it was the fact that I didn't have to fight to be heard, that people could see me and hear me and paid attention.

Everything was running like clockwork. I began to call the numbers, then ... to my horror ... I fell. The chair I was on had only gone and collapsed, hadn't it. And on cue, the entire hall erupted with laughter. I suppose it was quite a spectacle to behold. We know we shouldn't laugh, of course we do ... but we still do it.

Once all the laughter had died down there was an extremely uncomfortable and embarrassing silence. I was mortified. If I could have got up and run, I would have. Instead, I had to listen to it all and then wait until they decided to help. The attention was on me for all the wrong reasons, and I knew what they'd all be thinking: *He was too heavy for the chair, it collapsed under his weight and now he's paid the price by getting hurt.*

The manager rushed down to the stage. By that time, customers were congregating around me, pulling this way and that, trying to help but just making the embarrassment even worse. I told the manager to carry on calling the game. Of one thing I was certain – as soon as he called the next number, the customers would beat a hasty retreat back to their seats, their urge to win being much stronger than their desire to help me. My plan worked, though one customer remained and somehow (goodness knows how) she managed to roll me to the edge of the stage, enabling me to sit up. With a little further help from my friend, I was eventually pulled up and got back to my feet. As I'm sure you can imagine, by this time my dignity was in tatters. Nevertheless, I sat back down and carried on calling the numbers for the rest of the evening.

Each of these incidents had dragged me down further and made me loathe myself even more. I went home that night sore again. This acted as the catalyst for me taking time off work. What with the assault and falling off my chair, I didn't feel like I belonged there any-more. It was like the one place I felt I could be myself and be someone turned out to be a sick joke; another aspect of my life that I'd failed at. Then, because I was off for so long, I worried that I'd get sacked ... and then where would I be? You know what it's like when you start skipping doing something though, it gets harder and harder to go back to it and that was where I was heading. I must have been resilient to get this far in life though, must have been doing something right. All these obstacles would have finished many people off. But I was hurtling towards my threshold. Sometimes I felt I'd never got the chance to dust myself down before something else happened.

I think luck is very much a state of mind. If you think positively, then positive things are more likely to happen and, when they do, they boost you and lead to more positivity. When you are bombarded by negativity it is the exact opposite. You get lower and lower and can't see a way out, even reversing any success to fit in with your negative mindset. It becomes impossible to escape.

Just after my birthday in 2003, I was sitting on the settee in my living room, unable to move and very depressed. My legs were in so much pain that I could hardly sleep. It was three o'clock in the morning and I was watching a documentary about orchids. To be honest, I was hardly even bothered about what was on TV. But orchids? Who'd even want to make a documentary about them anyway? And what kind of sad audience would they attract at this time? Well, people like me, I suppose.

I really wanted to ring someone but there was no way I'd call anyone at such an hour. My legs were weeping so much that there was a massive puddle on the carpet where I was sitting. *I can't go on like this*, I thought. My legs were covered in huge ulcers, gaping holes oozed pus constantly and smelled rotten. It was like something out of a horror movie. I really wanted to end my life there and then but I just couldn't do it. If I thought I'd been low before, it was nothing compared to this. I didn't want to live anymore and I didn't want to die either. I'd sat so many times like this, and it felt like this was my very last time. I was weak, like I'd lost any fight I once had, like those were going to be my last moments.

I couldn't go to bed because, if I did, my legs would dry out and then tomorrow they would bring agony all over again and then would start to weep. But that's all they did anyway, that was the routine. I couldn't bathe them properly and so they'd be infected constantly too. I was even past the point of feeling disgusted with myself, my whole being was in pain both physically and mentally. I didn't feel all those other emotions, embarrassment, loneliness, distress ... it was like I'd submitted to all of it and nothing mattered anymore. Almost like being at peace with all the torment and torture and that I'd accepted that I was going to die. It was an odd sensation, though it was never a 'peace' in the real sense of the word.

I must have dozed off a couple of times and when it was time to I squeezed myself into a taxi and managed to make it to work. The shame of phoning up and saying 'It's the big fella,' the shame of putting my tea towel down on the seat before getting in, the shame of being out of breath after a few steps outside ... none of it mattered. I was on autopilot and didn't care. I would be safe and amongst friends at work and my good friend Lucy would look after me and have a look at my legs.

I arrived at work and, despite the fact I was in a mess, the customers always gave me a warm welcome and were pleased to see me. Gary and Marie were sat in their normal place, as were Mrs Ward and Philip, Cath, Audrey and my Marlene. They'd always be there.

As I spoke to Lucy, she said that one of the managers had asked her to have a word with me because he was concerned about my personal hygiene. This was something I was always concerned about too, but it was very hard for me – impossible, in fact – to be as clean and presentable as I wanted to be. I was very angry with him. Did he not realise how hard it was for me? Much of the bad smell coming from me was from the weeping dead flesh on my legs and under my stomach. I couldn't help that. I wanted to grab him and show him, make him understand some of the pain I had to live with.

Glenn, the general manager, was more sympathetic. He'd been concerned about the amount of time I'd taken off work and I know a lot of people thought it was only a matter of time before I went off sick and never came back. Lucy was one of the few people who believed that I would come through. When I used to phone in sick she would shout at me and make me come to work; she knew, as I did, that being at work was better for my mental and physical wellbeing than sitting at home.

Lucy was such a good listener throughout all this and helped me keep sane. In fact, she helped keep me alive. I know if it wasn't for her and her kindness I wouldn't be here now. Then one day she said something that took me by surprise.

'That's it,' she said. 'I am writing to Fern and Phillip at *This Morning*. I'm going to get some help for you.'

I didn't know what to say, whether it was an off-the-cuff statement or not. It was just left hanging in the air, really. But I kept asking her if she'd written the letter each time we spoke. I suppose I was goading her into doing it because I wanted her to. I worked with Lucy, and a few others had been part of the conversations, so it was all witnessed. She told me that she'd really fall out with me unless I did something about my weight because she was convinced I'd die. She obviously knew I was taking more time off than being in work and said she didn't want me to completely withdraw and sit alone at home eating myself into an early grave.

And then she did it. She wrote and sent a very moving letter saying that she was scared I would die and that the world would lose a wonderful man loved by thousands. She said she would rather see me lose weight than win the lottery. With the nation behind me, she said, I'd do it. It really hit home that she cared for me so much and wanted me to change. People at work said I still wouldn't stick at it. She told them that she believed I would and it was her belief that started to give me the kick in the pants that I needed. If someone had such faith in me, could I really fail? Or similarly, if someone put her neck on the line in such a way, could I break her heart by letting her down?

I was mad with her once she had sent the letter, but deep down I was excited about it. It was an odd mix of emotion: angry ... yes, happy ... yes, anxious ... yes, scared ... definitely. It felt like a real step this time, like I was finally able to admit to the world that I had a serious problem and I needed help before it was too late. In some respects, I already thought it was too late. I saw this as my last ever *I mean it this time*. It was probably on par with going to an addiction centre and announcing 'My name is Charlie Walduck and I'm a foodaholic,' only I was going to announce it on national television rather than to a roomful of people.

Of course, I was pessimistic about anything ever happening once the letter had been sent. And just to prove me wrong, the producers of the show rang me up just before Christmas 2003. To say I was slightly concerned about going on the show was a bit of an understatement. My nerves couldn't take it. But not only is Lucy a great friend, she's also very persuasive and told me I had to do it. It wasn't just friendship at stake here.

I said to Steve the producer that I would do it, but I wanted a say in how it would work. It isn't usually something that TV people agree to, but I asked if they'd not show any of it on TV until I had actually lost some weight. I didn't want the pressure of going on first, then having every man and his dog commenting, asking how I was doing, saying it didn't look like I'd lost weight or anything else. There were so many scenario possibilities that I needed to limit. People who knew me would obviously know what I was taking part in and that was fine. Another aspect I wanted a say on was some of the visuals they'd be shooting. It wasn't that I was being a prima donna – I just didn't want to be filmed eating. I've seen countless documentaries where the fat bloke says he wants to lose weight and you see him in cutaways shovelling food down his throat. I didn't want to be featured in that way because of public opinion and because it wouldn't have helped me at all. You wouldn't have seen an alcoholic necking a bottle of Scotch or a junkie shooting up, and I didn't think seeing me eating was that necessary. The producer agreed and I was happy to embark on the journey.

I'd been on dozens of diets in the past. And yes, they'd all been successful: I lost weight on all of them, but as you know, I never sustained it and put the weight back on soon after. Diets are usually based on the same basic principal: eat less and exercise more. I always did eat less for a bit and I never could exercise. And it was doomed from the beginning because I had no commitment.

Before meeting up, Dr Chris Steele phoned me to introduce himself and I was amazed. I didn't think it was him at first because he was a TV personality and it all felt a bit surreal. I used to watch *This Morning* and would switch the TV over a fair bit when he was on. It wasn't that I didn't like him, it was because I'd sit there and get paranoid about my health. There was a guy on once who had really sore legs through an infection and it was upsetting because it was just like the excruciating pain in my legs at the time.

When we met up, I told him that I did have an understanding of what a diet was and didn't want him telling me what to eat because I'd fail in a couple of weeks if I didn't like the foods I was supposed to live off. Dieting on something you don't like is never going to work because you'll never stick at it. And there are so many weird ones available to try, I can tell you. I know someone who tried the cabbage soup diet who didn't like cabbage and wasn't that fond of soup either. She didn't stick at it and never lost any weight before moving on to the boiled egg diet. She didn't like boiled eggs, loved them fried though. Then, to even the plate out, she'd add a sausage or two, some bacon, mushrooms to balance the meat out with some veg ... and before she knew it, she was on the fry-up diet.

I also said to Dr Chris that we needed to keep my diet simple. I didn't want to be stuck in the kitchen twenty-four-seven cooking and preparing food. It would be too difficult to do that because of my mobility and also because I wasn't brilliant in the kitchen anyway. I just wanted food with minimal fuss. I said I had a microwave oven and wasn't afraid to use it.

Anything like cooked meats, bread, cheese, yoghurt – anything that could be eaten without being prepared I couldn't have in the house and had to stop myself from buying it. I needed to have food that required some amount of thought to turn it into a meal or food that I just wouldn't pig out on, otherwise I would have been battling temptation from day one.

We settled on a plan: meals to contain less than three per cent fat and an eating curfew set at six at night.

'If it looks right and if it works, we will stick to it. If it doesn't, we'll agree to reassess and we'll get some other people involved to help,' said Dr Chris.

That sounded fair enough and it all moved along quite swiftly. As far as consulting my own doctor before going on a weight loss plan, I mentioned it, told him what I intended to do and he was fine with it. There certainly wasn't any panic. I mean, a forty-odd-stone bloke asking the doctor if it was OK to go on a diet sounds like the beginning of a joke, doesn't it? It was dangerous to go from 20,000 calories a day down to 1,500, but the way I'd been living was dangerous enough anyway. Each day I woke up could have been my last. There wasn't much to lose when you think of it like that.

My new regime was to have breakfast cereal on a morning with skimmed milk. I'd have this at home before going to work. And when I was at work, Beryl would bring fruit in for me for lunch, rather than us having the usual junk food fix. It was great that I had friends who were prepared to help. Even if they were not convinced by my dubious past attempts, I'm sure they were on their way to believing and wanted to make sure I gave it my best shot. Now, I'd still do my shopping online, but I'd buy low-fat healthy choice ready meals. I know these kinds of meals are constantly criticised for their sugar or salt content ... so hear me out. For me, they were portion controlled, cheap and easy for me to cook. I stocked up the freezer at home and at work and them being frozen meant I'd have to think about it before eating it, so it was on the 'safe list' of foods (i.e. not immediately edible). I'd have these for tea if at work and Beryl, bless her, would cook them for me. I made a note of everything I ate on a daily basis and it all went on a spreadsheet.

There would always be someone who'd suggest cooking a healthy chilli and freezing it. Well, I knew that cooking a huge pan of food would only lead to one thing. I just needed people not to interfere with their pearls of dietary wisdom and let me do it my own way. If it went wrong, then I'd take advice.

After filming schedules and other TV-land issues were sorted, the camera crew turned up in February 2004 for our first shoot. Deep breaths ... in through the nose, out through the mouth ... I'd have given anything to be anywhere else that morning. What I had to keep at the back of my mind was that it was going to change my life. I think that's why I felt such pressure; putting too much emphasis on it and giving it the all-or-nothing status could have been detrimental, though I'd defy anyone not to think like that in my shoes. There had been so much anticipation from that initial phone call, through Christmas, into the New Year, and then the date had finally arrived. It was like when you book up for a holiday months in advance and don't think about it until you have to find your spending money from somewhere by the following week.

They say that TV cameras make you look ten pounds heavier too. D'oh!

Weight Loss Diary by Charlie Walduck

So, there I was, ready for my television debut. There's a saying about 'bricking it' if you are worried. If this saying were true, I could have built a few bedrooms and a new dining room on to the back of the house while I was waiting.

Like many others, I'd cringed at reality TV and vowed never to do anything as potentially damaging to myself. And yet here I was opening the doors to television cameras in what was a first for the show and a first for me, of course. Once I'd said yes, there was no way I could just back out either. I'd made a commitment to seeing it through with regular filming to follow my progress. It was to be filmed over the course of a year, not just an insert showing me sampling a few salads for a fortnight and going back to pies after losing a couple of pounds. I was looking to lose the equivalent weight of nearly forty-seven large penguins, for God's sake. This was a serious mission.

It doesn't get much bigger than being on *This Morning* and I was determined that my waistline wouldn't either. I knew they were genuinely doing it to help me, but I'm not daft enough to think they were doing it *just* for me out of the goodness of their hearts. They were also doing it for the goodness of their audience figures, which is fair enough. Although I know there was no exploitation going on, whatever happened on my journey was sure to have enough drama to make good TV. I was fine with all that ... all or nothing. I was prepared.

Steve the producer phoned me on Thursday when he got to Manchester just to let me know he was there and all was well. I think it was to calm my nerves ahead of the shoot, and it did – until I put the phone down and it dawned on me. I was going to be on television!

The following morning was the one where I was bricking it. If I could have paced the floor with worry I'd have done so. As it was, I made do with tapping my fingers on the arm of my chair, channel hopping on TV, trying desperately not to think too much about it in case I backed out – all the usual things someone goes through just before making a fool of themselves on TV.

That was the point. No matter how good and positive I knew it was going to be, there was another perspective where I imagined what the viewers would be thinking. Would they laugh at and ridicule me? Would they pity or have empathy for me? At least by saying I didn't want to be filmed eating, I knew there wouldn't be as many 'no wonder you're so big' comments.

I was embarrassed that I was so big that I had to go on TV for help. It was like being fat defined me as a person: I'd become Big Charlie, the bloke who couldn't stop eating. No one saw me as anything else. Going on

TV was almost like going back to when the delivery guy brought his family round to see me ... morbid curiosity of the morbidly obese, only now the entire nation was being invited round.

As mad as it sounds, I breathed in a bit when I opened the door to the crew that Friday morning. I know it had no impact, but it was a natural mechanism – if the attention is on your belly, you breathe in to save face. And I was embarrassed about the state of my house too. Their visit had coincided with 'the maid's week off' and it showed. I'm pretty sure that they knew I was in no fit state to tidy up, so it would never have been an issue for them. For the crew, my house was a set that they had to light and film in. They really weren't that bothered about the tidiness as long as there was electricity, room to set up the camera and monitors and, most importantly, that I had a kettle.

One thing that wasn't shown on television was this enormous set of scales they brought with them that took the best part of the morning just to assemble. Steve the producer tinkered with them and got everything calibrated before I set foot on the plate. The problem was that an error message kept coming up on the display. It turned out that they only went up to forty-two stones and they wouldn't take my weight. Another set was sent down a couple of weeks later and I was able to get a reading at forty-four stone and two pounds. With this being nearly three weeks into my weight loss programme, it had been estimated that I was around the forty-seven stone mark at day one proper.

I kept a weekly diary during the entire process because I needed to monitor my progress. And I turned into a right geek with spreadsheets for everything: food intake, calories burned, where I walked, how long for, every meal and menu. Other than monitoring my progress, it was also compiled to help me spot anything I was doing wrong if the plan didn't work for me.

WEEK ONE
44 st 2 lbs

The camera crew left and I burst into tears. I felt so alone and isolated. Nobody had been in my house for such a long time and it was great to have some wonderful people caring for me. I hope I can do this. I'd been joking on with them all day, so when I said I was going to run the London Marathon in two years they all laughed. I was being serious about it! I know they'll not take it seriously at the moment though. They don't know it, but doing the marathon is my goal. Steve said he would do it if I did. I bet he doesn't!

I think that deep down Dr Chris doesn't think I can lose the weight. He's probably seen dozens of people half my size saying 'I'll start tomorrow,' so who could blame him? And following on from the filming, I had great supportive phone calls from him and Steve.

It is difficult to start something like this on a non-work day. I got back into work on the Sunday and everyone was asking how I was doing and I said I felt great – I've done a full day of diet, but nobody seemed impressed. I hope they are not expecting miracles, but it's early days. Dr Chris phoned Mum and she was delighted. She has told all the neighbours about it.

The first day was the hardest this week, but Dr Chris told me that the first day would be the hardest and that every journey starts with the smallest step. He also said this is the biggest I will ever be and my weight will fall off as I continue. I feel great.

I'm not sure what I was expecting to happen. There was nothing *to* happen, really. After all the build-up, there was the inevitable comedown. I cried bucket-loads; pure, pent-up emotion came flooding out. And once it was all out, I did feel good. It was like the first day of the rest of my life – a brand new start. I wiped away those tears, composed myself and phoned Mum and told her that the crew had been and gone. It wasn't that I was begging them to stay; I knew why they were there, I think it was more because of how it had made me feel. I was the centre of attention, in a good way, and this was quite a first. I wasn't a sideshow getting pointed and sneered at; people were asking me questions, listening to my replies and it was all interesting enough to go on TV. I felt special for the first time in ages. They'd been there from nine in the morning until nine at night, a long day for us all.

It did come with its downside though. Even in documentary-style programmes like this, you have to set scenes up to give an impression of reality because it's still a constructed story. That meant they had to film me walking to the kitchen, walking upstairs and whatever else to show what I'd be doing if the camera wasn't filming me (although I'd probably just be sat down all day). I'd generally only go upstairs once a day (when I went to bed) so this made filming even more of a strain. Sometimes I just slept sitting on my chair if I couldn't get up. The pain in my legs and knees from having to perform for the camera was excruciating.

Remaining positive through this wasn't easy but, because I could, I knew there was hope. The thing is, even if me walking to the kitchen was perfect first time, they would usually call this their 'safe take' and get another as backup so they had plenty coverage for when they went into the edit. If they don't have enough visuals, it either means a reshoot and more money or losing the shot or sequence, so I just had to go with what the team said and trust they knew what they were doing. Which they did.

I had a few ideas of how I wanted to come across, but back then I wasn't the media-savvy expert I am now. All I thought was that I'd answer questions, talk for an hour or so and then they'd screen it. Being edited means they'd pick out the best bits and can give their own 'spin' on the situation, to an extent. I don't mean this in the 'They did me good and proper – stitched me up like a kipper!' sense, just that I didn't know the process.

To get to forty-odd stone takes a hell of a lot of dedication and to lose thirty of it takes a whole lot more. At that point, all I was to Dr Chris was just another promiser. The cynical Mr Walduck just thought, 'Oh well, I'm never going to see him again' when he left my house, and he proved me wrong by phoning me on the Monday. He told me to write down how I was feeling and to put a spreadsheet together of all that was going on, what I was eating, what exercise I was doing and send to him so a record was kept.

I used to weigh myself on Saturday mornings and would ring Mum to give her 'the scores on the doors'. If it was a good week, I'd be so happy about it that when she asked for the 'scores' I'd be like, 'Have a guess, have a guess!'

The first few days of dieting were the worst. Obviously, no one was ever going to see a change in me within those days, but inside I could feel it. I knew I wasn't eating all the rubbishy foods I'd usually consume and I felt great that I was resisting the temptation. Man, this was a massive breakthrough and I wanted to run around shouting about it. You know, a day without crisps or a pastie for me was a miracle that didn't mean anything to anyone else.

I think my colleagues at work were rather sceptical. *He's on another diet? OK, we'll see how long this one lasts.*

I knew they'd be thinking these thoughts. What the hell. Stick at it. Show everyone what you are capable of.

I pre-warned them that on my birthday on 30 August I'd be having all the treats that I'd missed out on and for them not to give me a hard time because it would be a celebration, a reward.

He's making plans for August when it's only February. He'll never even last until March.

When the crew had gone I felt so low after the high, and that was when I'd usually turn to food. I didn't on this occasion. I'd taken that first step and couldn't wreck it all on the first night. This was going to be good, I could feel it.

Please give me the courage to be able to do this. Please don't let me mess up, don't let me fail. I'm a good bloke, really. I know that if I'm granted this one last chance, I can make good of it. You've got to believe me.

WEEK TWO
44 st 2 lbs (amount lost 0)

I feel as if I have eaten too much this week but I also feel as if I have lost some weight. I have had loads of calls from Dr Chris and support from the team at *This Morning*. Everyone at work is totally behind me and it feels so right. My legs are still very sore and I am having a nurse around every day to wash them and put bandages on. One of the nurses was very rude indeed. Some people are just plain horrible, even in the 'care' profession.

The nurse was so open with it. It was disgraceful. She'd been round previously in her 'nursing' capacity and I'd actually complained to have her taken off my case. As I started to lose weight, my legs still needed treatment and I still needed a nurse. I was dreading this woman coming round.

'I see you still haven't lost any weight,' she said when I opened the door.

I wanted to tell her where to go, to be as nasty as she was, get in her face and really show her what it's like to be bullied, but I've got more manners than she'll ever have. What a spiteful way to go on, eh?

To be a nurse, you have to have a bit of understanding and empathy. The world is full of people like her though. Luckily, I haven't encountered that many of them. I got used to the odd comment such as 'It doesn't look like you've lost much' or 'You can't have that because you're on a diet,' and it would have driven me up the wall if I'd let it get to me. There were a few times in the supermarket when, once someone had recognised me, they'd look into my basket to see what I was buying and then think they had the right to comment.

You know, I could easily have become aggressive, always on the attack, always snapping at people for no reason, if I didn't rise above it all. These were the smaller obstacles, but all the same, they were the ones that would niggle away at me when I had some spare time on my hands and when my inner demons were there to mess with my state of mind. Importantly, once the demons got me in their grasp, I'd start eating behind closed doors again. If these people knew the effects of their snide remarks, I'd like to think they'd keep them to themselves.

So, with my legs, Lucy had always been my carer and had done everything anyone could to help me. I went to the doctors and was advised to see the district nurse who'd apply treatments and bandages and whatnot, but I just couldn't physically get there. No one seemed to grasp this, but in the end they did, hence nurse sourpuss coming round.

At my lowest point, I wished I could just have my legs amputated and be done with the pain. I knew it was my own fault and certainly didn't want to be reminded of it by others.

This is it, Charles. This is it. Two weeks into a diet and already you're moaning and want to quit. That's you all over though, isn't it? If it's too much, just give up … make some excuses, tell a little joke and go back to eating. It's all you know. It's all you'll ever know.

Oh, woe is me. Isn't it terrible, having to eat normally?

It's pathetic. Re-educate yourself? Don't make me laugh. You've lost no weight and you never will. Get used to it.

WEEK THREE
44 st 2 lbs (amount lost 0)

I am into week three and I still have not lost any weight. HOW? It is so frustrating. I am feeling very low and not sure if I can carry on with this. I will hopefully lose some weight this week. I am eating breakfast every morning, fruit on my lunch break and a low-fat ready meal for my main meal. Surely this must be doing something.

Oh God, someone please help me. Three weeks of living like this ... three weeks. I made my promise. I stuck to it. I've done everything I should be doing. Why has nothing happened? What's wrong with me?

I'll do anything, give anything. I just want to lose weight. This body is killing me. I can't take much more.

Please do something.

WEEK FOUR
44 st 2 lbs (amount lost 0)

Nothing. Again. Dr Chris has told me to keep on doing what I have been doing, but I'm getting a bit bored with the diet.

Why did I do it? Why did I live like that? All the time I was shovelling food down my throat without a care in the world, was I actually thinking at all? Why the hell did no one stop me? What kind of person eats and eats until they're the size of an elephant and doesn't do anything about it? The only time I finally say I'm going to seriously do something about it – and go on national television to do it – and what? Not even half a miserable pound. I must be the only person in history to go on a diet for weeks, scrutinising every meal, every mouthful, and for what? Nothing, that's what.

All those times coming out of pie shops and feeling guilty, the looks from people in the street, the abuse ... all down to me and what I did to myself. It makes me sick just thinking about it. Why couldn't I just be like everyone else?

WEEK 5
43 st 9 lbs (amount lost 7 lbs)

Oh. My. God!

At last! I weighed myself today and I am pleased to say I have lost seven pounds. Seven pounds! I checked and double-checked, and double-double-checked. Seven pounds! I am feeling so much better about myself and feeling thinner too. Dr Chris, Steve and Natalie from *This Morning* phoned me for updates and I was so chuffed to tell them because I was beginning to think they thought I wasn't even trying.

Brenda at work has been great and she has said she will do as much as she can to help me. My legs are very swollen and sore and I have been struggling to get around. At work this week we were short staffed but I couldn't get off my chair to help and I felt very guilty about it. My friends Gary and Marie (bingo customers) have been really supportive too. It's great to know I have such good friends.

In discussing weight loss with Dr Chris, he put my mind at ease with regard to the initial disappointment. As I'd started my diet and hadn't been able to weigh myself until two weeks into it because of the error message on the first set of scales, he said that I'd almost certainly lost weight immediately during that period. When I did get the chance to weigh myself, it must have been after losing initial pounds and it was quite common to not lose any more for a few weeks after. So really, there had been no problem, it was all normal, I was just a bit out of synch with my weeks to begin with. It was just the kind of positive news I needed to get me really fired up.

At that early stage, it would have been so easy just to pack it all in. It was so demoralising to commit to it and to see no weight whatsoever come off. It was just ridiculous. What did I have to do to lose even a single pound? Run a marathon a day? It seemed impossible that I could make an absolute change of lifestyle and see no difference.

At just five weeks in, I used to think I couldn't face having the same food again. It was day in, day out low-fat ready meals fresh from the microwave. To stay motivated, and believe me it was difficult to stay on track at the thought of another shepherd's pie, I'd think about a conversation I had with a girl. She had lost a load of weight herself and looked amazing; it had been a real transformation she'd gone through and it had all been by sticking to a weight loss plan. I asked her how she kept going when she looked forward (or not) to the same meal for dinner, which she'd been having every day for a year.

'Nothing tastes as good as the feeling of being slim,' she said.

How cool did that sound? Maybe it should be attributed to someone else (she didn't come across as someone who spent her time postulating such QVC presenter-esque sound bites) but it was always something that would come back to me time and time again when piercing the plastic film on the ready meal packaging.

At around this point in my mission, I started to eat different foods. It wasn't a case of lapsing back into a bad habit, though: I created a new and better one.

Thursdays were my day off and I started to get a bit adventurous with my food. This didn't entail just sitting in front of the Discovery Channel while having a fish pie, but actually involved real cooking. I tried my hand at making a chilli and found that I had a real talent for it. If I'd tried that before starting my plan, I'd have shown my main talent and demolished the whole thing immediately. It was unusual for me to behave like this. I was well on my way to transforming myself and my mind. I was reconditioning myself through positive thought. I didn't need to eat everything in one sitting. The temptation was there, but if I kept the chilli, there'd be some for the following day. You have no idea how good I was feeling. Although I hope you do and I hope you have felt it too, because it was the best.

By making a chilli, I'd usually eat a bit more than my usual pre-packed portion, though it wasn't anything that would set me back. And having this as a weekly treat gave me something to look forward to. It gave each week a focus and broke up the monotony of 'same old, same old'. I'm sure pizza every single day gets boring at some point.

Did I just say that out loud?

WEEK 6
43 st 3 lbs (amount lost 13 lbs)

No, really, did I just say that out loud?

I weighed myself and I have lost six pounds in the last week. I'm very happy about this and feel very satisfied.

I had Yorkshire pudding and roast beef for my tea on Sunday. It was really nice but I thought it was a bit fatty. It was amazing that I could taste the fat on the roof of my mouth afterwards.

I seem to be moving around much better this week although my legs are sore and the nurse has given me some cream to put on them. I have been feeling a bit anxious too. I have another appointment with nurse next week and will also have my toenails cut. In terms of weight loss, I am feeling quite good. I am hoping to get down below the 600-pound mark when I weigh-in next (I'm currently 605). I have a tape measure now and will take a measurement and give details in next week's update.

I knew there were a lot of people who thought I couldn't do it. My track record at sticking to diets wasn't that impressive, so who could really blame them? I couldn't get bogged down with negativity though. Yeah, I knew I'd not stuck to dieting in the past, but I also knew that I had a 'do or die' attitude now. Once I saw the weight starting to come off I felt unstoppable.

Lap it up while you can. It won't last, mark my words. Losing a bit of weight ... so what? You've lost that before and it was back on quicker than you lost it. I know you too well. You'll never do it. Thirty stones? Now that IS funny.

WEEK 7
42 st 9 lbs (amount lost 1 st 7 lbs)

The weigh-in: fantastic news! I have lost eight pounds in the last week and I am so very happy. I'm working tonight, and to top a good day, Barrow FC won too! I can't wait to feel mentally and physically fit enough to go to a football match again.

Took my waist measurement at seventy-eight inches. It was

about eighty-four inches when I started. A loss of six inches! Feeling really good this week. My legs still feel terrible, but they cannot dampen my spirit.

WEEK 8
42 st 0 lbs (amount lost 2 st 2 lbs)

Wow, another nine pounds lost in a week. I can't believe it! I feel amazing today, on top of the world.

We had a quiz on Sunday of this week at work and they put a big buffet on. Pork pies, sausage rolls, sandwiches and savouries – all my favourites – and I never had any of it. And I won the quiz as well!

I have had the nurse round every day this week to treat my legs and they have got much, much better. I've been to see my doctor this week and she was very supportive about the weight loss project. I made an appointment because I've been feeling a bit stressed of late (I can't imagine why!) and she gave me a leaflet about coping with panic attacks, etc. Producer Steve e-mailed on Sunday, Dr Chris on Tuesday ... both pleased with my progress. I hope I can keep it going – it's the weigh-in next week. Fingers crossed!

WEEK 9
41 st 9 lbs (amount lost 2 st 7 lbs)

Another five pounds bites the dust. I'm pleased with this but I would have liked to have lost a bit more. I'm on a roll now and not even a sausage in sight. It's mad that I lost five pounds and feel I could have lost more.

My legs are still quite sore and getting me down, but they are feeling better than they were. I'm concerned that I'm not walking enough at the moment; this will come in time. Lots of articles and stuff in the papers this week about obesity and get-fit campaigns.

It would be great to think that I can be a positive role model in eighteen months to two years' time. I want to show people that there is no such thing as 'the point of no return'. You can always turn your life around if you want to. I've not done it yet but I am so determined this time. I tell myself every day 'you are fitter today than yesterday and tomorrow you will be even fitter.'

Next week I am off work for almost three weeks so this will be a real test of my willpower.

Looking back at my diary, it brings back the feelings I had at the time. It's like reliving it. To have been that size, becoming that size literally all my life and having to live with it – to see it starting to drop off was the biggest high. It was fuelling me to carry on: with each pound I was losing, I was saying goodbye to a body I hated being trapped within.

It also reminds me of the trouble I had with my legs and knees. I still have the scarring on my legs as a constant reminder. They had been under so much strain for those years and it's a wonder I hadn't done permanent damage to them; just the cosmetic shame I now suffer.

WEEK 10
41 st 1 lbs (amount lost 3 st 1 lb)

I have weighed myself and I am delighted I have lost eight pounds this week. I am thrilled by this. I am moving around much better. I know I tend to repeat myself and write the same every week but this is how I feel.

I know I tended to repeat myself and write the same every week, but that was how I felt.

Week ten already? Three more weeks and I have done a quarter of a year. I am going to take my scales into work soon and I'm going to do a weigh-in every week with some of the customers. I am going to try and organise the diner at work to do a healthy special and we are going to have our very own diet club every Sunday lunchtime. I announced this week's weight to the customers this afternoon and got a big round of applause. It was amazing. I'm hoping to drop at least another stone while I'm on holiday. Steve and Dr Chris are coming to visit next Saturday.

You just need to go back a few pages and it is like reading the outlook of two different people. I was on the brink of giving up everything not too long ago and here I am saying I want to lose another stone while on holiday. I mean, holidays were usually a time to wallow in more self-pity and overeat; a time for sitting in front of the TV for the duration and spending all my money on having unhealthy food delivered.

At ten weeks in, I really was a different person. I had a purpose, I had a goal and I had the support of people to help me along. I'd always have my dark moments and periods of doubt. My depression was never going to just get up and leave because I lost some weight. It's never that easy. Having fire in my belly rather than a load of pasties was a good feeling and I had a fighting spirit. I knew I could fight the inner demons and I knew they could easily win battles if I let my guard down. Because those demons are 'me', that's what makes it all the more difficult. Your demons know all your weaknesses.

WEEK 11
40 st 10 lbs (amount lost 3 st 6 lbs)

A loss of five pounds over the previous week and Dr Chris and Steve were here to witness it. It has been such a busy week this week. On Wednesday afternoon I went and had my hair cut and got stuck in the chair. It was something to laugh at rather than feel embarrassed about because I knew that a few weeks ago I wouldn't have even made it to the barbers, never mind fit in the chair in the first place. I went to a quiz at Belle Vue dogs that night and it was really enjoyable. Thursday was a long day spent with Steve and the crew. It was nice being with them and it was easy to forget that it was 'work'.

I bought a new pedometer from eBay and I managed to break it after just a day, so my step-count is still guesswork. Since starting the 'plan' I have lost forty-eight pounds, which is three stones and six pounds and represents 7.77 per cent of my original weight.

On Thursday, going to Barrow was very stressful for me, just getting on a train for the first time in years was very hard. I was being followed by TV cameras as well.

'Is it Brad Pitt?' I heard one lady ask.

Yeah, he spends all his Thursdays in Barrow, did you not know?

I got on the train and someone asked if it was one of those fancy tilting trains. *It is now*, I thought as I stepped on. At the end of the day the crew left and went to Barrow for a pub meal. I really wished that I could have gone with them. Maybe next time. The next couple of days at Mum and Dad's is going to be tough because I know their kitchen will be well stocked. They have gone away and I am looking after the dog. I would love to try and take her for a walk while I am here.

WEEK 12
40 st 2 lbs (amount lost 4 st)

I lost eight pounds this week, which is another amazing result. Steve from *This Morning* rang and I was telling him I felt like I was being re-born – like a plant that had not been watered for ages and was being to grow again.

I have lost fifty-six pounds now, which is more than a sack of spuds! And the percentage now lost is 9.09 per cent of my starting weight. I have been on the scales every day this week, which is probably not the thing to do, and I don't seem to have done very well. The pattern seems to be eight or nine pounds one week then five pounds the next. I went to Morrisons supermarket for the first time in two years as well this week. I am so very proud.

WEEK 13
39 st 8 lbs (amount lost 4 st 8 lbs)

Another eight pounds bites the dust. I ate my first bread in three months this week with my lunch on Wednesday. It was really nice. It really gave me the taste for it. I used to eat a lot of bread. Maybe better off steering clear if I can.

When we get to the end of this week then it is actually thirteen weeks since the start, which is a quarter of a year. I went to Carpet World on Monday afternoon to buy a rug for my bedroom. I am really starting to take some pride in my home and trying to take some pride in myself also. This is a good sign because I never had any pride for either in the past.

My waist measurement on Monday night was taken at seventy-three inches. It's reduced by eleven inches since I started. People are starting to notice that there is something different about me, finding it hard to determine exactly what. When I see that quizzical look on people's faces, I know I'm making good progress. It'll soon click with them immediately.

WEEK 14
39 st 5 lbs (amount lost 4 st 11 lbs)

I walked around the block this week, thought I was going to collapse when I got back, had to stop and sit on someone's wall for a few minutes (I hope they don't need to rebuild it!). I could only manage it once, but every little helps doesn't it? I only managed to lose three pounds this week but that's OK.

When I started my BMI (Body Mass Index) was eighty-seven and is now down to seventy-seven. To achieve a safe BMI, I would have to be thirteen stone. Just twenty-six to go, then! My pedometer entries are estimated this week as I need to get another new one, as my last took a swim down the toilet. Have been reading some interesting things on the *This Morning* website about 'good' foods, turkey being one of them. I always thought turkey was foul though (get it? Foul/fowl? I know, don't give up the day job).

BMI stands for Body Mass Index and is the measurement of fat in your body. Nearly all of us have a set of scales and nowadays they can be quite technical and give us all sorts of information about our bodies. It is important to always use the same scales every week, weigh in the same place and wear more or less the same clothes. I always weigh naked on a Saturday morning. I have had some funny looks in Boots I can tell you! When you are trying to lose weight, the temptation is to step on the scales every day, and I'd be a liar if I said I didn't get tempted, but try not to because it really can put you off.

BMI is quite complicated to work out to say the least (weight divided by height squared), but you can find BMI calculators all over the interweb.

Categories of BMI:
    18.5 and below means you are underweight
    18.5–24.9 is normal
    25–29.9 is overweight
    30 or above indicates obesity.

WEEK 15
39 st (amount lost 5 st 2 lbs)

The hot weather is playing havoc with me and I have terrible 'nappy rash' at the moment. I'll have to stop wearing nappies soon – see if that helps shift it. When I get down to my marathon weight, things like nappy rash will be a thing of the past. I was very sore on Wednesday and Thursday this week with it and was a bit low as a result.

My mum and dad came round on Thursday which was really nice. I filmed my mum talking about how I am doing. We went for a short walk down the road but it was hard because my legs were really sore. Natalie from the show rang me the other day for an update, which was nice, and she was really impressed with me ... she said she is going to do the marathon as well!

I wasn't really wearing nappies. I meant that my legs were rubbing together and with such heat it was an absolute nightmare and I needed to bathe as much as possible.

WEEK 16
38 st 12 lbs (amount lost 5 st 4 lbs)

I only lost two pounds this week and I am very disappointed. I did a piece-to-camera and I was so upset. On top of that, my legs are still sore. I don't know if I can carry on but I will keep it going for now. Feeling desperate.

Had my shopping delivered on Wednesday. Have bought some Sultana Bran because I am not going to the toilet as regularly as I used to and I think I need a bit more fibre in my diet. Last week was so bad weight loss wise I decided to weigh myself every day this week to see where I might be going wrong (if indeed I am going wrong). By Wednesday, I was six pounds down on the previous week and then by Wednesday night I was only two pounds down on the previous week, so I have knocked that idea on the head.

Got a new pedometer from Steve at *This Morning*. My average steps now are about 1,000 a day; it was only 400 when I started.

WEEK 17
38 st 2 lbs (amount lost 6 st)

Lost ten pounds in the last week – fantastic! I have also increased my steps this week and the daily average is now almost 3,000.

One of my main rules is to not eat after 6pm but when I got in on Sunday I had one of my meals. I couldn't stop myself and this worries me. I suppose this is my first slip even though it's just a little one.

This was a dark time for me. I was gutted that I'd broken one of my rules; it was something I couldn't get out of my head. The main worry was that if I could break the rule once, I could easily do it again, and that would see me lapsing back into my old ways. I was also still a bit down from the previous week and these were the things I was trying to get rid of from my life:

negative thoughts and eating at the wrong time.

I'd made too much progress to throw it all away. If I didn't let go of the negativity, I'd sink back and I knew I'd start to eat again, convincing myself of failure.

So that was it. I regretted it, hated that I'd done it, but I had to move on. If it was so easy to lose weight, I'd have been able to do it long ago. I just needed to stay focused. It was a tough job and I was the only one who could do it.

What did I tell you? I knew it! Can't do it, can you? I knew you'd never last. You never do. This is just the start.

WEEK 18
37 st 13 lbs (amount lost 6 st 3 lbs)

Only three pounds lost, but on Friday I walked the most steps I have ever done since records began ... 4,400!

WEEK 19
37 st 9 lbs (amount lost 6 st 7 lbs)

Four pounds. Average steps 3,300 a day. Not too shabby.

WEEK 20
36 st 11 lbs (amount lost 7 st 9 lbs)

Unbelievable! This week I managed to lose twelve pounds! That's like the weight of a dog! Maybe more ... a big dog? My legs are still sore but, despite this, I did my most steps ever on Tuesday, managing 4,600 in one day.

On Thursday I caught a bus for the first time in three years. Three years! The price of a ticket had certainly gone up considerably, which was a bit of a downer. I sat at the bus stop and, as I looked around, I could see loads of other people totally unaware that I was having difficulty just being there. Getting on the bus was a right struggle and a half. I had to let two buses pass before I eventually had the courage to get the third. I felt proud of myself, but at the same time very frightened. Not sure I will be able to do it again for a while – I started to panic a bit when I got into town. I had to meet Joanne, Brenda and Zeta from work to look at some Christmas stock for next year. It was hard work and they carried a chair around so I could keep sitting down. Beryl from work has been walking me around the car park. I'm hoping to be able walk a bit further soon.

One thing that Dr Chris said to me was that I needed to exercise. I needed to start walking. My reply was that I couldn't make it from one side of the room to the other in one go, but he told me I had to start doing it. He'd given me my first pedometer and I did 300 steps on my first day and vowed to increase on a daily basis. Pedometers had a very limited life expectancy with me and I knew I had to step up a gear or two.

Beryl and I took a trip round the car park at work one day and we increased that to walking round the building, to the bus stop and pretty soon I thought that if I could make it to the bus stop comfortably, there'd be nothing to stop me getting on a bus more regularly than once every three years. You need goals to keep you motivated. The same thing each day gets too boring for someone like me.

When I told Dr Chris I was walking, he agreed to come round every Thursday on his day off. The first time, we literally only managed a few meters before I started struggling. I was short of breath, sweating and needed a sit down. If I were in Dr Chris's shoes, I'd

121

have been wondering what the hell I'd let myself in for. Our walks round the block took twenty minutes and, at one point, we passed a group of kids who I was certain would shout abuse but we got by without incident. Safety in numbers!

Thursdays were great – we'd walk and talk and he never questioned what I was eating because he could see I was doing the right thing. The results were visible. My plan was working and didn't need to be altered. I'd also have less than the allocated 1,500 calories if I could.

Progress with walking was slow, but it was progress. We kept going a little bit further each week, making sure everything was achievable; nothing too silly. That was the key. Do what you can and don't kill yourself by doing an extra few steps. As I built up these walks with Dr Chris, I gained enough confidence to go without him. I was keen to prove to myself I could do it. Going out alone was something I'd never have thought possible before starting the weight loss programme and was another great confidence booster.

We got to the stage where I would go over to see Dr Chris if he couldn't make it to my place and the conversations were no longer based around food. It had become a proper friendship.

Once we were out together and were stopped by a man on the street who was keen for a chat. He said how great it was that we were out exercising. 'You must be proud of what you've done, helping him lose all that weight,' he said to Dr Chris.

'No. I'm proud of what *Charlie* has done. He's done it all, not me. He's the one who has had to live with it all this time. I'm just here once a week,' he replied.

I knew he understood, but hearing him say it meant a lot to me. It made me proud to have such a mate.

WEEK 21
36 st 3 lbs (amount lost 7 st 13 lbs)

Eight pounds. This is just bizarre. This is now the longest diet I have ever been on. Most steps ever on Friday, 6,300. How good is that? Ian Botham eat your heart out!

WEEK 22
35 st 13 lbs (amount lost 8 st 3 lbs)

Lost four pounds last week.

Wednesday: I cooked turkey breast in chilli with two jacket potatoes. It was far too much, but I hated to throw it away, so I ate it all. I feel bad about it. Very bad. When I was eating it I felt as if I was slipping back into my old ways and, for a few moments, a kind of mist took over my body and I wanted to eat everything in sight. It was horrible. I felt really out of control and it scared me quite a bit. This is exactly what they mean by 'falling off the wagon'. I did resist everything humanly possible after that moment though. I weighed myself on Thursday morning and it seems I have lost NOTHING this week yet. I'm a bit disappointed about this, but am now back on track and staying positive about the weigh-in on Saturday. On Thursday I went to Morrisons for a look around. I did my most steps ever on Friday this week, almost 9,300.

Nine thousand three hundred steps! Who'da thunk it, eh? It felt great to be able to just go out and walk somewhere, like a miracle had taken place. I used to envy people who could walk and used to know that, deep down, it would be something I could never do. And now I was walking freely wherever I wanted and doing things I hadn't done in years. I was determined not to start taking walking and catching the bus for granted. When you've lived without something for so long, it is impossible to imagine having it back. To me, it was like a fresh start. Like when you learn to ride a bike as a kid, you want to go everywhere on that bike. That was me with walking. I couldn't understand why people would want to drive to the shops or get a bus into town.

Oh, another slip up? That is good news. Don't think that going for a walk will make it any better, because it won't. Let's see how long it takes for the next one.

WEEK 23
35 st 10 lbs (amount lost 8 st 6 lbs)

I lost three pounds last week and I am now down to five hundred. I'm really craving pies and pasties this week. I literally can't stop thinking about them. I dream about the food I miss, almost to the point of thinking my duvet is pie crust and I'm in a giant pie, eating my way out. I could easily eat my duvet if I'm not careful.

I do feel positive and, as we move to the six-month mark, I think my progress has been remarkable. Not blowing my own trumpet or anything, but I mean, eight and a half stones is the weight of another grown person! I've lost a person in weight! I know that if I want to sustain this forever, then I need to re-educate myself and come up with a plan for the rest of my life. The only way that this will work in the long run is if my life changes and I can continue on my fresh start in terms of everything I do in my home, social and work life.

My average daily steps are now close to 5,000, which is half what is recommended. I need to do more!

I will always be prone to weight gain because of my

addictive personality. Much like depression, it's always going to be there, following me around and waiting for me to slip up. Other than my life changing, I need to do it the active way, rather than passively. I need to change my life, not hang around waiting for it to happen.

WEEK 24
35 st 3 lbs (amount lost 8 st 13 lbs)

Lost an amazing seven pounds last week, meaning that twenty per cent of my start weight is now off.

On Tuesday night a narrow-minded customer said something very insulting to me about my weight. It upset me because I can't understand why people feel they have to do this. Are they so insecure that they have to insult others to feel better about their own lives?

On Wednesday I had some visitors round, but in the morning before they came I was very depressed and low. I don't know why and later I felt better. I did a lot of walking on Wednesday too. I did the duck walk (not a duck in sight) in the morning then went to Newton Heath market, Morrisons, Asda, the antiques place and the catalogue bargain shop – loads of walking. The duck walk is so named because there should be some ducks around by the water. There never are. It's still going to be the duck walk though. I'm sure one day I'll see one.

On Friday I am seeing a counsellor at the health centre; I'm trying to sort myself out mentally too. I need to start to build my confidence and not worry so much. I need to learn to like myself. I am feeling quite low this week so I am looking forward to the chat.

I always get embarrassed talking about growing up, shaving and being a man. Especially in front of Mum and Dad. The counsellor said this was maybe down to something traumatic happening during adolescence where I'd put a hold on certain feelings and I hadn't actually fully gone through the adolescence process. I can't think of anything or maybe I blocked it out. Maybe being overweight meant I didn't experience adolescence until I'd lost it all. There was never any interest in chasing girls, playing football, driving cars or anything else that lads growing up have an interest in. We all know my interest by now.

When I'd been to counselling in the past, probably a year before, to talk about my concerns, it had been a case of getting a taxi to the health centre that was literally just round the corner, then getting up a couple of flights of stairs when I got there. It hadn't been worth my while at all. Having to get a taxi somewhere that you could probably hit by throwing a stone is not very good for your self-esteem. If it wasn't so obvious why I needed a taxi, I'm sure the driver would have had a go at me for going on a journey that didn't even require second gear.

I think it may have been the armed robbery that led to me going to talk to the counsellor, because of the downer that I was sent on from it. The robbery left me shaken and I felt like a real victim for quite some time after. I thought seeing someone and talking about it might help me to forget about it, put it to bed and move on. Having to walk up the stairs though was practically impossible for me. It made me feel worse about myself, going to see someone and not being physically able to make it to their door.

WEEK 25
34 st 11 lbs (amount lost 9 st 5 lbs)

Lost six pounds last week! What's that? The weight of a cat? Not quite as good as losing a dog's weight, but a cat is not to be sniffed at. Especially if you have allergies.

When I weighed myself last Saturday I was delighted because for the first time in ages I weighed less than my age. This felt like a massive milestone for me; a personal goal achieved. I always used to joke when I was a twelve-stone twelve year old that I would weigh fifty stone by the age of fifty. I almost made it there before the age of forty. That's pretty bad. I need to keep what Dr Chris said in mind – I will never be that big again.

I am on holiday next week and I need to start to plan what I am going to do to fill the days. I am going to try and find something to do every day so I'm not tempted to sit at home and eat. Duck walk: where the hell are the ducks?! If I don't see any soon, I'll have to call it something else. They must see me coming with a loaf of bread and hide, thinking I'm coming to make a sandwich.

Ten things that have changed:
1.   I can walk more
2.   I can put my hands behind my back
3.   My watch is loose
4.   My shoes are too big
5.   I can clean myself a bit better
6.   I can fit in chairs
7.   My clothes feel better
8.   I wore underpants for the first time in ten years
9.   I sleep well every night
10.   I fit into the toilet at work

Seeing these changes was amazing. You know, most of these things are experiences that I'd never had. I'd only ever been able to fit into the disabled toilets at work because the doorframes had been modified and were wide enough for wheelchairs. I'd never been able to find underpants big enough, my shoes were a size too big because my feet were fat and I could actually reach parts of my body now to clean. It was unreal. I could never transpose that kind of feeling on to the page.

WEEK 26
34 st 4 lbs (amount lost 9 st 12 lbs)

Lost seven pounds this week. Next week it will be my official six-month weigh-in and would be great if I was to hit the ten-stone mark for the occasion. Not to *be* ten stones – I mean to have lost ten.

WEEK 27
33 st 8 lbs (amount lost 10 st 8 lbs)

The official six-month mark and I am delighted to have lost more than ten stones. I lost ten pounds last week! Me, Charlie Walduck, losing ten stones in six months. No one would have believed it was possible. I should have gone to the bookies six months ago and put a few hundred quid on the big fella. In all seriousness though, ten stones in six months is pretty much impossible. If I can do so well in half a year, I can do the same in the other half.

Last week was a stressful one and this week has been too. It was my birthday on Monday and on Tuesday my Auntie Margaret was taken ill. It is very difficult being off work. If I'm not constantly occupied, I'm risking turning to food. A lot is happening this week. I can't believe it is six months since this thing started. In some respects, it's flown over, and in others, it has dragged out. I've seen such a dramatic change in every-thing about myself and I'm muchos chuffedos about it. I've been as low as I always used to be and have come out of it each time unscathed. There's been one or two times where I've overeaten that I'm not happy about, but what can you do? At least I didn't lose the plot completely and ruin all the progress I'd made.

It turns out that blueberries are the new 'super food'. Dr Chris recommended them and I bought some at Morrisons. Can't say I liked them that much. They taste much better when surrounded by muffin. A mate of mine said blueberries are 'a bit pointless' as they don't taste of anything, and I'm beginning to believe her. I estimate that I have walked nearly nine miles this week. It's like being back in the Sunday Club!

I used to hear people complaining about how difficult it is to lose a few pounds. There'd always be someone somewhere who would come out with a ridiculously long sigh, followed by 'I'm depressed' or 'I'm fat.' I used to cringe. It was like they'd be gloating or were probably too dumb to realise they were saying it in front of me. It was generally for attention that people would say that, fishing for compliments and wanting someone to say 'You're not fat, you're gorgeous.' I'd just lost nearly eleven stones by putting my mind to it, not eating too much, eating less fat and walking. That's all. It was no big million-dollar secret. It would be great if people thought before opening their mouths, but some people can't. I really hate the 'I'm depressed' line. You just don't say it if you are depressed or if you've experienced any kind of mental illness. I don't know ... some people, eh?

Half-time break

I f someone was to pass me in the street at this point, which they did, they'd still stare at me. Which they also did. At thirty-three stone, I was still a big bloke and still struggled to do things. A six-month success was only part of the journey. I mean, it was still front-page news that I could walk anywhere and do things because most activities were physically taxing for me.

One of the biggest changes I made eating-wise was breakfast. Before starting my weight loss plan, I either didn't eat breakfast because I didn't have time, or I ate a few breakfasts in one go. There was never a happy medium. And not having time is just like saying you don't have time to walk to the shops ... all you need to do is schedule an extra twenty minutes or so and it will set you up for the day.

If you're serious about losing weight or just wanting to be healthy, the best way to start is by having a good breakfast. Any time I have skipped brekkie I wanted mid- or late-morning snacks, and that's where the big problem is. A balanced breakfast can also provide the right vitamins and minerals to kick start your metabolism and make you feel awake and alert and ready for your day. I know that sounds like something from a healthy eating leaflet, but it's true. Those times when I just got ready and went to work left me starving all day and I was also a lot slower and took forever to wake up properly. We live in busy times where we need everything in an instant and we live at a fast pace. If we started to think more about the fuel we need to do this, we wouldn't skip meals and wouldn't need daily fixes of energy drinks and fast food. I'm sure there are many of you out there who can relate to what I've just said, and really, all this is about is common sense and looking after yourself properly – something we're all capable of doing.

Breakfast is a meal; that's something we tend to overlook too. It's like we feel guilty for having something substantial on a morning, going for something substandard instead. I mean, is a slice of toast going to fill you up and provide the right energy to keep you going until lunchtime? Would you have a piece of toast for dinner? I think the sooner we realise that breakfast is the most important meal of the day then the sooner we'll be able to live with having more than two mouthfuls of food without feeling ashamed.

It's also common sense that if you have a big breakfast you have the whole day to burn it off. A good friend of mine once told me that she struggled to lose weight and that she never ate, but simply snacked during the day. When I suggested she wrote down everything that she ate, she was amazed by how much she actually consumed. I told her she needed structure and every structure needs a foundation and our food foundation is breakfast.

Never forget that you have a choice of what to eat.

It isn't just bird seed for breakfast and rabbit food for lunch, you know, and it is worth considering what is out there and doing a bit of research ahead of devising a plan. There are loads of choices when it comes to breakfast and, like with everything else, we are faced with a series of healthy or unhealthy choices to make: will I lose weight by having cereal or wholemeal toast rather than a fry-up? Is a full pot of coffee with two sugars in each cupful good for me? Is it wise to lean over the bed and start eating the takeaway from the floor first thing in the morning? Hopefully, these are all common-sense answers.

Look out for wholegrain cereal as it is widely publicised that it is good for the heart, and skimmed and semi-skimmed milk will help you reduce the calories. A good serving of milk each day on your cereal will give you much of your daily calcium requirement as well – it's a win–win situation. As an alternative to milk, I sometimes use yoghurt or add fruit whether with milk or with yoghurt. Bananas are great with cereal and will go towards your five-a-day fruit intake, as well as containing three natural sugars: sucrose, fructose and glucose, great sources of energy.

Toast can be wholemeal bread with low-fat spread rather than white with lashings of butter; breakfast on the go can become a muesli bar (look out for low-calorie ones) rather than a McKentucky King fast food solution or greasy sarnie from a van. If you are accustomed to the Great British Fry-up, try toning it down a bit and replace the bacon for turkey rashers, sausages with Quorn ones and boil, scramble or poach your eggs. Don't fry anything: use the grill instead, it's much healthier. Eggs are packed with a range of nutrients including protein, essential vitamins A, D, E, and B groups as well as minerals iron, phosphorus and zinc.

They're relatively low in saturated fat, containing around eighty calories each, so they are eggstremely good for you. And they are not eggspensive (I'll stop now). In fact, if you've got a hen, they are completely free.

Beans are cheap as chips! Maybe the wrong simile to use there but you can get cheapo tins of beans in most supermarkets for less than ten pence these days and you can do loads with them. They can be used as part of breakfast, lunch, dinner – whatever – and even the skins are full of nutrients. Just watch out for the salt and sugar levels in them; this will be listed on any tin and most places do a healthy option version these days. They are exactly what you have bean waiting for, and no kitchen cupboard should be without a load of tins.

Oats are oatso very good for us and have been around since the beginning of time. They contain soluble fibre that helps to lower cholesterol levels and keep you feeling full for a long time afterwards. Good old-fashioned oatmeal porridge will provide you with an excellent slow-releasing carbohydrate. This is another versatile one and is worth experimenting with by adding to it: chopped almonds for your good fat and protein, and sliced sultanas can be used to sweeten it. Or you can soak them in soya milk overnight, mix in sunflower seeds, add dried fruit and some more soya milk to taste.

In short, oats rule, but it is also well documented that we don't seem to bother with them that much. Recently, it's been said that oats can: help hangovers, help you stop smoking, fight infection, heal the skin, fight heart disease, slowly reduce diabetes risk, beat depression, prevent constipation, cut childhood obesity, boost energy, fight osteoporosis, help dieting, reduce blood pressure, help longer life, fight cancer, be good during pregnancy and improve your sex life. I'm not sure I can testify to all of them, but surely you oat it to yourself to give it a go. That kilt-wearing shot-putter on the cover of the box didn't get in the shape he did by necking fry-ups every morning, did he?

Of course, milk goes hand in hand with porridge and oats and is a great source of protein, vitamins and calcium. When I first started with my weight loss plan I really did have to re-educate myself. As I say, you cannot jump into something like that without doing some background research, and finding out facts about food was quite refreshing. As a child, we were always told that the cow juice was good for us and encouraged to drink it at school to go towards our recommended daily calcium intake, but it was only when I looked a little bit further that I found out all the positives. The one we're always told is that calcium is good for bones and teeth, but it also helps to regulate muscle contraction so is good for your heart and is said to help reduce high blood pressure and protect against some cancers. You also get calcium from green leafy vegetables such as broccoli, turnip greens, Chinese cabbage, cauliflower and salmon, tofu, almonds, Brazil nuts and dried beans.

A glass of skimmed milk measuring around 200 millilitres or so contains approximately 73 calories compared to full-fat milk at around 128 calories, but the amount of calcium provided is more or less the same.

As I've already said, one of the worries for me was that I'd get bored easily of the same food each and every day. In what seemed like no time at all, my mind was wandering and, when that happened, I knew I was in danger of eyeing up other foods. It's the same with anything once boredom sets in, so you need to spice things up a bit. Try warm milk on cereal in the winter, try a new variety of cereal when you start to wake up on a morning wishing you had something else to eat, try adding some exciting extras to your porridge. And some cereals contain essential Omega 3 fish oil, which means they are much better for you than a bacon and fried egg butty on a morning (mmm ... with tomato sauce). Or if you can be bothered with picking all the bones out and can put up with the after-smell in the kitchen, you could go to work on a kipper. Just make sure you keep a tight hold of it.

Healthy eating is not about punishing yourself, it's about reconditioning and finding out what you like. Don't eat the wrong foods at the wrong time and wonder why you're not losing weight. Although I always say it is a simple plan, you still have to go about it the right way and there's still a certain 'science' about it. The big thing for me was getting myself up out my chair and starting to walk. That was my big step, but my first smaller step was to start by having a balanced breakfast, which in turn was part of a planned weight loss programme.

You just need to type 'breakfast' into t'internet to see the amount of facts it brings up, such as 'Research has shown that a child of twelve that skips breakfast in the morning has the mental agility of a seventy year old in the classroom.'

When you see facts like that, it makes breakfast all the more important. Without a proper start, kids' ability to learn at school is limited and as adults we're not functioning to the best of our abilities either. We supposedly burn fewer calories through the day if we skip breakfast regularly, and regular breakfasters are less likely to suffer colds, flu and other respiratory tract illnesses than daily dodgers are. Presumably, this is because breakfast boosts your immune system. And by eating breakfast regularly, you are less likely to be emotionally distressed, depressed and to die by suicide, and you are four times as likely to win the Lottery and marry a supermodel.*

All you need to do is make the time. It is a very minor change that can have a major impact. The ingredients are not mega-expensive and the benefits are amazing. The one big temptation I had was not too long ago when listening to Radcliffe and Maconie on the radio. A bloke phoned in with a claim that he'd invented a breakfast pie. Mark and Stu were as stunned, as I was. A breakfast pie? This was like the Holy Grail of blokishness! I defy anyone who heard that broadcast not to imagine the biggest, most unhealthy fry-up packed into pastry, coming out the oven golden brown. Sorry to have put that in your mind, but breakfast pie! That is a genius idea. If there's ever a low-fat one, I want it.

Lunch, just like everything else in my life, also lacked structure. If I could have gotten away with it, my entire day would have been lunchtime. There was no regularity, no set time ... nothing. And, when I did eat, there was no moderation. As a child there was structure, but as I started to grow up (and out) that structure disappeared slowly but surely.

My new rules meant that I ate at the same time, had quite a grasp on controlling my portions and ate food with a certain fat content. I'll not lie – cutting

---

* It's worth pointing out that some of these facts are 'said to' have that effect and a couple have been completely made up.

down was an absolute nightmare. And like any addict, I can and likely will fall off the wagon at any point in my life. It's something that I'm prepared for. Off days are allowed as long as they don't overtake and your life becomes one long one.

If you forget to make your own lunch to take to work, there's always the temptation of buying the wrong food. We look for something easy and something where we don't have to think, and this is where fast food 'restaurants' cash in. Avoid going anywhere where they want to supersize you, as that's what you'll become, and avoid eating pre-packed sandwiches all the time. I used to think that the best thing to put into a sandwich was your teeth, but even I can be wrong sometimes.

Avoid the ones with loads of dressing because there is no such thing as low-fat dressing. Some products claim to be 'light' or 'diet', but those words have no legal definition. Try sandwiches made with low-fat meats and salads, try wholemeal bread or wraps or wholemeal pitta bread. There was a TV documentary on where many high-street chains were slated for their food's salt content. I'm not saying that they were right or that it was balanced in any way, but one chain came out on top and, if any, that would be the one I'd buy from. Then again, if you take the time to make your own and consider the ingredients in advance, you'll be saving a lot of money too.

It's quite common to think salad as soon as you think diet. If that's you, avoid those with too much dressing. Many supermarket salad bowls are laced with calories and a high amount of fat. For instance, a 300-gram bowl of shop's-own coleslaw contains around about 750 calories.

One of the easiest things to do if you are sat at a

desk working all day is to snack. Especially if your job is as boring as some of the jobs my friends have. And snacks are generally not good for you, unless you plan them with fruit, fruit salad, dried fruit or maybe a few nuts rather than a chocolate bar or something like Maltesers that you'd have one of every few minutes. Don't be deceived into thinking that snacks are OK simply because they are advertised as being lower in fat or calories. In my experience there is no such thing as a low-fat biscuit. And don't forget vegetables can be turned into a snack too. It doesn't take long to turn a carrot into carrot sticks. It costs a couple of pence and you can crunch away all day. Try the same with celery. And pea pods, when in season, are the best snack in the world ... you can even pretend they are miniature green Maltesers, if that helps. Just don't go dipping them in chocolate.

A friend of mine always eats his sandwiches at his desk half an hour before his official lunchtime. Then, when lunchtime hits, he's out on a walk for the best part of an hour and gets back to the office for some fruit and water before his break is over. A good thing with working in offices these days is that they always have water coolers. If your place of work has one, use it to get your daily intake. Fill a water bottle up before you leave and drink on your way home. Some call centres even supply free fruit because they know the positive impact on productivity.

Dinner, or tea if you're not as refined as me, is often the main meal of the day and, for many of us, it normally signals the end of a working day and a time to relax, unwind and catch up with family.

At forty-four stone it was difficult for me to stand in a kitchen and prepare and cook a meal. And without going for the sympathy vote, living alone meant that no one else would offer to do it for me. My dinner was usually a variety of unhealthy options from the shops near the bingo hall or an unhealthy option from the diner there. Either way, it would almost always include loads of crisps and a few cakes. I'd be sat down all the time at work and would ask people to fetch food for me if they were going to the shops or ask them to bring a burger or fishcake from the diner for me to snack on. It was textbook-style unhealthy living, and, of course, rounded off by junk food from the garage on the way home before a takeaway was delivered. When you can't cook, the easiest option is to have it delivered. In my case, though, I was having enough food for four people delivered.

When cooking from scratch, I try to go for low-fat meats. Turkey and chicken are both low in fat and can make a large number of meals. Quorn (the meat alternative) is also very versatile and can be used in a variety of meals. It is also very filling and surprisingly tasty. There are some veggie products that literally do look and taste like cardboard, but it isn't my place to go bad-mouthing them in print. Diets are not about eating something you can't stand even if it is better for you. Look around, see what's out there. Cut any visible fat from meats and boil or bake potatoes rather than having chips or roasting them. I tend to put jacket potatoes in the microwave first, then crisp them up in a pre-heated oven. There's always the temptation to whack a load of butter in, so go for low-fat spread or maybe baked beans to add something moist to the plate. Fish and vegetables with jacket potato is delicious too. I try to have vegetables with everything and always have water on the table and drink plenty of it.

On With the Show: Charlie's Weight Loss Diary, part deux. We rejoin Slimmer Charlie as he gets to:

WEEK 28
33 st 3 lbs (amount lost 10 st 13 lbs)

I went to Oldham Hospital on Monday for blood tests and chest X-rays. It was as bad as I imagined and now all I have to do is worry about getting the results.

I also went to Barrow this week and found it much easier than before and I'm sure I will be able to do it again soon. Something like this, just the thought of having to go anywhere, used to grip me with fear. Now it's an adventure. I like getting on trains and buses to go places and am so glad that I don't have to get a taxi and take my tea towel with me. It was a bit early in my progress to be going to Barrow but I wanted to visit my Auntie Margaret in hospital. She was so pleased to see me and it was nice to see her. She didn't look well and I'm hoping she will be better soon. It's never nice visiting anyone in hospital, but you always have to remember it brightens their day up if you do.

I did loads of steps again this week (my average is now 6,861 a day) and I'm moving about much better this week. I walked to the barbers for a haircut and it was hard work walking around ... and it was shut. Typical!

I'm having an ECG next Monday and then on Wednesday I have an appointment with the doctor. I don't know how much more of this kind of fun I can endure. I'm not really a big fan of anything medical, even *Casualty* on a Saturday night does my head in.

I've done almost nine miles again this week. Not bad at all.

WEEK 29
33 st 1 lb (amount lost 11 st 1 lb)

Only lost two pounds this week so I was a little bit disappointed, but all weight loss is something and I need to keep that in mind.

Blood tests: the doctor said all my tests were normal apart from two of them. The ALT [a test that detects liver injuries and disorders] was up, but Dr Chris said not to worry about this as it was likely due to having a 'fatty liver'. Also BSR [which indicates inflammation somewhere in the body, likely due to wear and tear on the joints] was up.

Quorn: the advertising campaign for it is to 'Try it – you might be surprised,' and I must admit I was surprised. It mustn't have taken long for them to come up with the strap line for it; I could have given them that one for the price of one of their cottage pies. It was really good and I will definitely be having it again. Very nice indeed. Only 4.2g of fat for the whole thing and only 174 calories. The only problem: not enough in this 300-gram pack for me.

Dr Chris wrote to my doctor to ask if he'd send me for medical tests. I later found out that he thought I'd have all sorts wrong with me, such as diabetes. Then there was the problem with my legs; I was terrified that I was going to lose them. They stunk so badly of ... well, of death. It was like they were dying from the abuse they'd endured and if I went for any tests I knew this would be discovered. All my anxieties from my self-diagnosis resurfaced again. I reluctantly agreed to tests as long as Dr Chris agreed to accompany me.

When the day came, Dr Chris couldn't make it, so I had to go to Oldham Hospital on edge and on my own. When I got there the lift wasn't working and I had to be on the third floor. It was a miracle that I made it alive, to tell the truth. Walking was bad enough, but going up flights of stairs really took its toll on me. If I didn't have a heart problem previously, I was certain I'd have one after getting to the top. Medical tests were supposed to assess your health, not add to your health problems.

As an added poke in the eye when I finally made it, I was too heavy to get on to the table for a full X-ray. They managed to X-ray some of my joints, including my knees, and I was told I had arthritis in them. A blood test turned out to be fine, blood pressure fine, cholesterol fine and I didn't have diabetes. However, my liver appeared to be functioning abnormally and I had to take a bucket away with me to wee in for twenty-four hours (not non-stop, don't be silly). Actually, when they said I had to urinate in the container for twenty-four hours I did think they meant non-stop at first and couldn't help but have a chuckle as my mistake dawned on me. I'm sure they were used to the reaction. I had to tip some of it out in the end. I could have easily filled another, grabbing an old KFC bucket out the bin and sticking a bit of cling film over the top: 'Here you go, doctor. Not at all. Don't mention it.'

It seemed I waited for ages to get the results back. Convinced it was going to be cancer, I phoned Mum to blurt out all my anxieties again.

'It must be cancer,' I said. 'I'm losing weight and everything.'

'Don't be so stupid, son. The reason why you're losing weight because you're on a diet,' she replied.

She had a point there.

Eventually, the results came in and showed I had Gilbert's Syndrome. I've no idea who Gilbert is, but his syndrome cannot be treated. Thankfully it isn't life-threatening.

When Dr Chris saw the results, he said 'Charlie, I don't understand it. You have none of the diseases that are associated with obesity. It doesn't make sense.'

Other than a bit of wear and tear on my knees and a common liver complaint, I was medical science fiction and very relieved about it. If my weight had also been down to drinking or if I'd been a smoker, then I certainly would have had a load of health problems.

The embarrassment of taking my clothes off in front of someone, feeling like the Elephant Man and the indignity of being examined were the reasons behind never wanting to seek medical advice in the past. Being there in Oldham was because I had to. I'd lived in fear of surgery for such a long time and knew that if I did need any kind surgical procedure then I may as well wave goodbye because I wouldn't survive it. I was too heavy to come out the other side cured: people my size don't. I didn't want to die having a routine operation, and you never know when you're going to need one of those. Any stomach pains I had, and I endured a lot, I immediately thought it would be appendicitis and I knew I wouldn't pull through if that was the case. I always just took the blokey 'It'll be gone in a week' approach to any ailment.

When I discussed my concerns with Dr Chris, I mentioned the time I'd been put under general anaesthetic when I dislocated my shoulder. He told me it could have been fatal. Back then I probably weighed around thirty stones and the hospital should have known the danger. I've fallen over in the street since then and dislocated it again. I fell in Bolton (why is it always Bolton?) where I had five people trying to pick me up. A shopkeeper brought a chair out and it took forever to get to my feet. Talk about embarrassing. I was so angry with myself in situations like that. The anger was that I'd let myself get so big that I couldn't even do a simple thing like get up off the floor – so heavy that I couldn't lift my own weight. I went to the hospital after that fall and the nurse said 'You know, you're going to have to lose some weight, Charlie.'

If there was ever a call for a 'No shit, Sherlock' reply, that was it, but I just told her I was well aware of that fact. The thing was, at the time it happened, I actually had been losing weight.

WEEK 30
32 st 10 lbs (amount lost 11 st 6 lbs)

I lost five pounds last week, really happy with this. That's 160 pounds lost in 29 weeks, so it's an average of over 5 pounds a week. Morrisons have brought a new range out called Eat Smart, they are healthy option ready meals with less than 3 per cent fat and around about 300 calories per meal. I tried the curry and rice and it wasn't too shabby (seven out of ten).

When I was in Morrisons on Monday I bought pizza for Beryl for her tea as I always get her something for tea, and one of the women who works there said, 'You can't have that!' I explained it wasn't for me, but I don't think she believed me.

Not the best saleswoman in the world, eh?

On Friday I did a massive 11,234 steps, which is fantastic. I started by walking to Morrisons, then caught a bus to Manchester and did some shopping. And while shopping I bought some socks and shoes ... Me, in socks! And what's more is that the shoes are proper lace-up ones, not slip-ons. I couldn't even reach my own feet for years and now I'm buying footwear. It's unreal. From there I got the bus to Belle Vue and walked into work. I am so proud of myself. Over ten and a half miles walked this week.

It was great actually going to a supermarket and being able to walk around. Yes, I'd still get the odd dodgy look (and comment from the staff even), but it didn't put me off. I'd always read the food labels and choose foods with less than three per cent in fat; three grams per one hundred.

A mistake to make is going shopping without a list. All you do then is impulse buy and that is not good at all. If you're anything like me, you'll just walk aimlessly up and down the aisles and pick up whatever catches your eye, no method, no reason, no structure. If you've planned your meals in advance, you'll know what you need and you need to stick to the list. Oh, and do not go shopping when you are hungry.

Sometimes it is best not to take a trolley because you resist the urge of filling it unnecessarily. If you shop day by day, you can always get more walking in while you do it. Try getting one piece of fruit or veg you haven't had before each week, too.

WEEK 31
32 st 1 lb (amount lost 12 st 1 lb)

Another nine pounds. This is one aspect of dieting that I'll never tire of – the scores on the doors. I really can't believe it. I thought, and I know Dr Chris did too, that I would have slowed down or even stagnated by now, but it's still happening for me. Let's not tempt fate.

It has been a fairly sad week this week as my Auntie died on Tuesday. The funeral is on Friday and I am going to Barrow-in-Furness for that. I loved my Auntie Margaret and she was always kind to me. I know she would want me to do this and I am more determined now than ever. It has been very stressful and exhausting ... maybe one of the hardest weeks so far on this thing.

On Thursday I went to see the doctor with regard to the test results. Everything is OK apart from my BSR [Blood Sedimentation Rate] and my liver function tests. I will be seeing a consultant, but the doctor thinks there is nothing to worry about and it is just a formality. The ECG was fine and normal. X-rays: fine apart from a bit of wear and tear in my left knee, which will get better with more weight loss.

Auntie Margaret had been in hospital after a blood transfusion where she was given the wrong blood type. It was one of those things that didn't have to happen and it was such a tragic waste. It was sad and it hit everyone hard. She was ace, my Auntie Margaret. She had such a tremendous sense of fun, just completely off the wall, and she was very kind. Some days, she'd watch the weather forecast on TV and if it was raining in Scotland she wouldn't leave the house because of it. I got on really well with her because I think we shared the same sense of humour, always wanting to find a laugh in anything.

WEEK 32
31 st 11 lbs (amount lost 12 st 5 lbs)

Lost four pounds last week.

On Wednesday this week I decided to treat myself ... not with food but a trip out to Blackpool on the train. It was a fantastic day and it was also hard work. I went with Gary and Marie, regulars and good friends from work, and we had a great time. I don't think I've ever gone to Blackpool and not enjoyed myself, it's one of those places that has that effect on me. The rides, the lights, the shops, the scale of the place ... like Blackpool was built around the idea of having fun. We played bingo and won a couple of times and walked along the sea front. The step count was over 15,000 after hoofing it up and down the promenades and beach and I think it will be a while before I hit that mark again.

On Thursday I felt stiff and sore but it was well worth it. Marie suffers from anxiety really badly and she was panicking sometimes and so was I, so Gary had to put up with the both of us. We went to see a fortune teller just for fun and she said I had an exciting year ahead and that I would have twelve children. Not sure what her day job is, but she shouldn't hand her notice in.

My average steps now are 7,500 and it won't be long before I get myself towards the magical 10,000 spot.

WEEK 33
31 st 4 lbs (amount lost 12 st 12 lbs)

Seven pounds lost last week! Waist down to sixty inches. I'm the incredible shrinking man!

WEEK 34
31 st 1 lb (amount lost 13 st 1 lb)

Lost just three pounds in the last week. At work loads of

customers are commenting about the weight loss. I am feeling really good and my steps are now an average 8,500.

WEEK 35
30 st 8 lbs (amount lost 13 st 8 lbs)

Another seven pounds off last week, and:
1. Caught a bus home at night
2. Went to Barrow to see Mum and Dad
3. Visited my sister in Ulverston
4. Managed to get a seatbelt on in Dad's car
5. Walked to and from station to Mum and Dad's house

WEEK 36
30 st 9 lbs (amount lost 13 st 7 lbs)

I put a pound on and walked almost thirteen miles.

Let's not dwell on it. One lousy pound, for goodness' sake.

WEEK 37
29 st 13 lbs (amount lost 14 st 3 lbs)

I am back on track with a loss of ten pounds. I also did 16,000 steps in one day last week and my average steps were over 10,000. Dr Chris was as relieved as I was.

WEEK 38
29 st 9 lbs (amount lost 14 st 7 lbs)

Four pounds ... *ker-ching*!

WEEK 39

29 st 3 lbs (amount lost 14 st 13 lbs)

Six pounds. Nice one.

WEEK 40

28 st 11 lbs (amount lost 15 st 5 lbs)

Another six pounds. Had a really busy week this week. I went to a bingo day out with the customers on Sunday, which was really nice and had a few nice comments from people who had noticed that I have lost some weight. It was a lovely day, but I was sad when it was over. On Tuesday I went to Morecambe and met up with my mum and dad and we took some pictures at the Eric Morecambe statue and had a nice day walking around the shops. On Wednesday I had to go the doctor and got some good news as the doctor was really pleased with my progress. On Thursday Dr Chris took me down to Granada TV as he was on a TV show and I got to see behind the scenes.

WEEK 41

28 st 5 lbs (amount lost 15 st 11 lbs)

Six pounds again.

Dr Chris wrote to me: 'I just want you to think about all that weight you've lost. All that fat hasn't been cut out of your body – it's been burnt off as fuel for your energy needs, purely as a result of your increased exercise/exertion. So it is vital that you concentrate on doing more exercise or the same exercise done at a quicker pace. What another brilliant week!

'As you say you have now lost 15 stones 11 pounds and you are certainly on target for losing 16 stones by Christmas. So for goodness' sake keep walking as much as you can in the next fortnight, so that you can walk off that 3 pounds, just to be able to boast that you have certainly lost 16 stones before Christmas. You must work, or walk, towards another 3 pounds' weight loss.

'Your next target is the 12-month target, which is only 12 weeks away, but I have to be honest that your target of losing another 59 pounds, to hit the 20-stone mark by then, is pretty extreme – it's an average of 5 pounds every single week! But at least give it a go!'

WEEK 42
28 st 4 lbs (amount lost 15 st 12 lbs)

I only lost one pound last week so I am a little disappointed with that, but a pound is a pound so it's better than nothing. It could have been worse – I might have gained. Mum and Dad came for two days and we went to the Trafford Centre and also went to see a show. It was good. The seats in the theatre were really tight, but I'm still a very big guy and am just trying to take it one day at a time. It will soon be Christmas and that is going to be a *very* big test. Average steps now are almost 15,000 a day.

WEEK 43
27 st 9 lbs (amount lost 16 st 8 lbs)

Nine pounds lost in the last week. Get in! I am so happy about this. I have another busy week this week so I am hoping and praying for more of the same.

I have now lost an amazing 231 pounds (462 blocks of butter!). It was the Christmas party for the customers this week and I was Santa. I went with Beryl from work for a Christmas meal out and it was great to forget the diet for a bit and just enjoy being out without feeling everyone was watching what I was eating, and be relaxed.

We also had a staff night out at Belle Vue dog track and there was a quiz night on too. There was a big girl there called Tracey, from Liverpool. I said hello to her and then my friend Shaun came out with a dodgy comment when her back was turned.

'She'll not be on the quiz team; she'll only be here for the free buffet.'

I was stunned. That was the kind of comment I'd always feared, the reason why I'd stay at home rather than eat in company.

'Shaun,' I said. 'That's not nice at all. Just 'cos she's a big girl, doesn't mean she deserves that.'

I turned back to her, 'All set for tonight then, Tracey?'

'Nah. I'm only here for the free buffet,' came her reply.

You could have knocked me down with a feather. What a laugh we had, but at the comment, not at her expense. Good on her to say it.

WEEK 44
27 st 7 lbs (amount lost 16 st 10 lbs)

My weigh-in was on Christmas Day. I probably overate today but I avoided cakes, sweets, pastry, bread, fried food and other festive favourites. I originally intended to have a feast day, but one is never enough and I was scared what it would lead to. I lost two pounds in the last week, so I am pleased with this. I helped out today at the Salvation Army in Failsworth. I've always wanted to do this and it was very rewarding.

I found an old pair of jeans in the cupboard, size fifty-four inches, and I managed to get them on. They were a bit tight, but I can say I had skinny jeans long before any of the Emo kids did.

Christmas past: could hardly move; just sat down and ate and ate and ate and ate, my house a mess, my life a mess.

Christmas present: enjoyed the build-up, the shopping and doing all the stuff normal people do. It was a bit lonely and quiet, but this year is a period of transition for me and next year will be better.

Christmas future: hopefully much happier with family and friends, all enjoying Christmas and everything that comes with it – and doing a proper job that will give me time off!

WEEK 45
26 st 13 lbs (amount lost 17 st 3 lbs)

Eight pounds lost in Christmas week. How often does that happen?

WEEK 46
26 st 5 lbs (amount lost 17 st 11 lbs)

There goes another eight ...

WEEK 47
26 st 2 lbs (amount lost 18 st)

Three pounds in the last week – not exactly up to Walduck standards, but I have now lost an incredible eighteen stones and I can hardly believe it. I'm keen to lose twenty stones by the time I have done a full year, so I have six weeks to lose twenty-eight pounds.

WEEK 48
25 st 10 lbs (amount lost 18 st 6 lbs)

Another six pounds down. If I wasn't living through it and

seeing it happen, I'd think it was a lie.

WEEK 49
25 st 7 lbs (amount lost 18 st 9 lbs)

Three pounds this time.

WEEK 50
25 st 7 lbs (amount lost 18 st 9 lbs)

I didn't have a weigh-in this week as I was at Jackie's wedding. It was nice seeing all the family, including Auntie Doreen and Philip (my cousin) and Steve and all his family too – seemed like ages since I'd seen him. I felt really good and took loads of pictures. My face looks bad; I have a lot of spots at the moment and feeling very conscious about this, but I am very much a 'work in progress'. I just need to concentrate on the future.

WEEK 51
24 st 11 lbs (amount lost 19 st 5 lbs)

I have started to go swimming now and on Wednesday I managed to swim seventy lengths. I did feel very embarrassed when I first went to the pool but once you are in nobody can see.

Dr Chris sent me a great e-mail: 'What great news, that you've now lost 19 stones 5 pounds. Now the target you have to get in the next two weeks is a weight loss of another 9 pounds, which means you will achieve your own target of losing 20 stones in your first year.'

WEEK 52
24 st 3 lbs (amount lost 19 st 13 lbs)

At the end of this week I will have done a whole year. Last week I managed to lose eight pounds and so I am just one pound away from losing twenty stones in a year.

One year ago, I could hardly walk. I was spending £100 a week on taxis and £100 a week on takeaways. Things have certainly changed in the last year and I now have some wishes to add to my list:

1. Learn to drive
2. Go abroad
3. Find a new job
4. Go to the football again
5. Get myself some kind of social life

WEEK 53
23 st 13 lbs (amount lost 20 st 3 lbs)

It's the one-year anniversary of the start my weight loss plan today. I weighed myself this morning and I'm pleased to say that I have lost four pounds in the last week, making a grand total of twenty stones and three pounds in the last year. My weight is now twenty-three stone and thirteen pounds. As a surprise for losing so much weight, all the production team took me to see Barrow AFC play Stafford Rangers. It was wonderful and we had a great day. Even though Barrow didn't win.

Everyone was coming up to Dr Chris at the game and asking him for his autograph.

'What you doing here?' someone asked.

'I'm a Barrow fan,' said Dr Chris.

I felt so very proud.

We went to a restaurant for a nice healthy meal and

some great conversation. All of which was condensed to a minute or so of screen time. After that evening it was over, it was a wrap. The entire process was shot and in the can and it was back to normality, reality and the comedown that would follow.

I went home and, as you probably have guessed, started crying immediately. I couldn't believe it was all over.

B   ack to life, back to reality, the song goes.
    And that's how I felt. I was deflated, a bit
    miserable ... it was a huge comedown. It had
    all ended. A year of being on top of the
world, of seeing all that weight come off, and now
what? Back to sitting in front of the TV?

The following week I only managed to lose two
pounds and felt devastated by it. If ever there was a
time for a shoulder to cry on, it was now.

I turned to Dr Chris and he wrote the following
letter to me:

'First of all, I thoroughly enjoyed the match at
Barrow. It wasn't such a bad result, 2–2, and, although
it's only a small ground, the enthusiasm of the home
crowd was very impressive. Isn't it great to see such
commitment from the supporters who have obviously
been through "thick and thin" with their local club?

'So, you only lost 2lbs last week – that's great, but
unfortunately you've set yourself such high standards
that you become disappointed with what is regarded as
a good weight loss. Even if you lost only 2lbs every
week for the next 52 weeks, you'd end up losing
another 7.5 stones! Everyone going on to a weight loss
programme is told that, at best, they should expect no

157

more than a 1–2lbs weight loss every week. Your problem is that the "Charlie Walduck Diet" has so far produced results far in excess of that. You've become your own severe taskmaster, expecting too much, so take heart, you are doing fabulously well.'

It was nice to hear these words and it spurred me on. Dr Chris had been a GP for over forty years when he read the letter Lucy sent in. He'd seen common colds, kids getting peanuts stuck up their noses and hands superglued to broken plates, but he'd never seen anyone lose thirty stones. At the time we started, I just assumed they'd read Lucy's letter and gave it a yay or nay, though that was far from the case.

Firstly, a meeting was held at *This Morning* and attended by all the top brass. Dr Chris advised that extreme weight problems are always difficult and he said they should find out a bit more about me. From there, he said he'd assess me and, if OK, they'd give it a try. If I'd known all this was going on in the background, I'd have been even more terrified. It's quite a daunting feeling to have TV producers and experts discussing you in meetings. It wasn't just about 'Can he lose weight?'

Knowing my story wasn't being broadcast straight away and the fact that I might not achieve the goal limited their responsibility. If it all went pie-shaped, then it was an experiment that didn't work and they weren't obliged to screen it. If that happened, then no one would have known anything about it other than us who'd filmed it and the odd person who'd heard about it. The only story would have been another failed attempt at losing weight because I lacked the will-power to follow it through.

Dr Chris wouldn't have agreed to me doing it unless he thought there was a slight chance. We'd spoken on the phone and he knew I was of sound mind and raring to go. They'd have massive reservations, of course I knew that. They'd have discussed me and my mental health, wondering how someone could get to where I was and how it had impacted on my state of mind, the way I functioned as a person ... everything, really. I could have been an absolute maniac for all they knew, getting to that size by roaming the countryside on a night eating cows and sheep. Who knows?

Another factor is production costs. It isn't cheap to send a camera crew from sunny London up to rainy Manchester to film something if there is no intention of it going on air. So it must have been a reasonable proposition, even if they knew it was a big challenge. Dr Chris also living in Manchester was another swaying factor for them. It was a great coincidence for us, but if we'd lived in different parts of the country I doubt it would have gone ahead because of the contact and support I needed. It would have been a logistical nightmare because Dr Chris used to come over to see me on his day off and there's no way I could have expected him to do that if I'd lived anywhere outside of the same city. At my weight when we started, there was no way I could have travelled anywhere to meet him.

I suppose they also had an ethical dilemma to think about. For all I knew, people may even have been inclined to complain to the show or the regulatory bodies claiming that I'd been exploited. Again, this was why they needed to know that I was aware of what I was doing and understood all that was about to happen.

Dr Chris is always keen to point out that he didn't feel pressured by the process. The process was all down to me: the pressure, the hard work, commitment.

Everything that happened happened because I did it. I'm certainly not bragging by saying that, what I mean is I needed people like him behind me for support. Just knowing he was there if and when I needed him was enough to keep me motivated; knowing he was on my side and was only a phone call or short journey away filled me with confidence. His son is an Olympic athlete, so he's seen firsthand what it is like for someone to commit to exercise. He's watched his son gobble down 6,000 calories a day and burn it off through training, and he saw me doing the same but without the burning off. There's no escaping the exercise – you cannot lose weight without that element.

As the filming process was coming to an end, there were some journalists sniffing around, asking if there was a guy going on TV who'd lost a load of weight. There was panic at the studio because if the press got hold of the story and ran with it, they'd ruin the whole thing by jumping the gun. There wasn't long to go before broadcast and it was a bit of a weird time. It would just take one person to mess it up by spilling the beans on the whole operation.

Also as we were getting to the end, the crew were round filming one day and I had the TV on. *This Morning* was on and there was a trailer for me on there! How strange did it feel? Very. It came across to me as quite 'tabloidy' and shocking and I told them I didn't like it. I was worried that my segments would be edited in the same sensationalist style and it would all look wrong when broadcast. I was assured that this wouldn't be the case. They said, 'Don't worry. Everyone will love you.' I can't imagine anyone not worrying.

Up until then, it hadn't seemed that real. I knew I'd been filmed, but my whole focus was more on losing the weight and I'd grown so used to being filmed it was something I stopped being conscious of. Actually seeing some of the footage for the first time made me realise that there was another goal – I'd been living it and the crew had been documenting and telling it. Their goal was to film me and put the story together in a balanced way. My story. That was another surreal one. My story now had changed from 'Hugely Overweight Man Struggles to Get By in Life' to 'Man Who's Lost Twenty Stones in the Space of a Year Now Has a New Lease of Life and a Second Chance'. Good things like this surely weren't supposed to happen to me. I wasn't used to such positivity. The five films were edited, we had transmission dates, I knew when I was to appear live on the show ... it was as real as it gets. The work was over. Time to enjoy the achievement.

My story started in April 2005, on Monday, and the films were to be screened over the course of the week with me being in the studio on the Friday for the big finale. The first one was the introduction and, natu-rally, it had to set me up as a big, overweight man who was depressed and couldn't move much. As my wish had been granted, I wasn't portrayed as an overweight man who sat eating and wondering why he couldn't lose any weight. There were *a lot* of tears in that first film. It was painful for me to watch, but that was because I was bearing my soul on TV. It was powerful, wasn't tabloidy and was certainly not something you'd watch and ridicule. The second film wasn't that uplifting either, although they did start to get more positive. The tears were all pure emotion. It was me being me and telling the world what it was like to be me. There was no acting.

I had a call from Lucy just prior to the third one

being shown. Something was up. She was a bit shifty and asked if she could come round to see me. Mum had been a bit odd around the same time too and I knew something wasn't quite right. Lucy came round and we watched the show together. For this episode, unknown to me, they'd interviewed Lucy, Mum and Dad, Jackie and my brother-in-law with head-and-shoulder shots of them all saying how well I'd done and how proud they were of me. They'd even filmed the taxi drivers saying well done and wishing me luck! It was amazing having people who were proud and wished me well. To see that happen on TV is something else.

I travelled down to London early on the Thursday and met Justine at the studio before being introduced to Phillip and Fern. Phillip shook my hand and congratulated me and Fern gave me a big hug. They said they couldn't wait to have me on the show, and just before the trailer for Friday's show they even said 'We're going to meet him later, but you'll have to wait until tomorrow.' It was great that they were so supportive and the way it had all been presented and followed up really involved the audience and made them feel part of it too. I never try to get overwhelmed by meeting famous people these days. The first time I'd had proper contact with a celebrity other than a quick photo or autograph was with Dr Chris, and now he was a friend. Meeting Phillip and Fern was one of those moments where I just wanted to point, scream and shout 'It's Phil and Fern!' And they were so down to earth and normal and I couldn't wait to get back there the following day. After meeting them, I went into London and did all the touristy things you're expected to: covered myself head to toe in Union Flag clothing, went on an open-top bus, went to Buckingham Palace, got crapped on by pigeons in Trafalgar Square and got confused by a the map of the Underground. I did it all. I also phoned Mark, telling him where I was and what I'd been up to.

'I'm in London.'

'What are you doing in London?'

'I'm on telly tomorrow. I've been on all week. Have you not seen it?'

'Eh?'

'I've lost a load of weight.'

Talk about surreal. Other than me saying I was going to be on TV, the losing weight bit must have sounded like a practical joke.

'That's mad. I'm in London too,' he said.

And it turned out that he was literally a stone's throw away from me as we were talking, to the point where we could almost have heard each other without phones. It was so good to talk to him after losing touch for a good year or so. We met up for coffee and had a right proper catch up, vowing to keep in touch properly after that. Makes you wonder how you can lose touch with people so easily.

I was at the studios on Friday for the show going out live and it was the biggest response they'd had for a guest in its history. There were phone calls and piles of e-mails. I cracked a few jokes about takeaways in my area closing and taxi drivers' car maintenance bills going down and it was such a great time. I felt so relaxed and on form. It felt quite natural for me to be in front of the camera. I know I had been for the past year, but a studio situation to a live audience is different: there's no 'cut' and 'let's go again' opportunity, no seizing up when asked questions, no cups of tea and no casual swearing to be done. Bah, live TV, eh?

Then they showed a film of everyone at the bingo

club cheering for me! The crew had shot this on the Wednesday that Lucy had come round; another reason for all the shiftiness. And then the tears started again. It's so difficult to put into words – going through that process, all the soul-searching, the highs, the massive lows, the daily struggle, training my mind to readjust, pushing myself to the extreme and never giving up, the anguish of not losing any weight at first, the thrill of losing several pounds a week and the changes my body and mind went through. Doing this and being filmed, achieving my goal, proving to everyone that I could do it, proving to myself that I could conquer anything and then it all coming to a conclusion live on television with all your closest friends who were on the journey with you cheering and praising you ... Well, I think I can be excused for shedding a tear or two.

And straight after the final episode, Phillip Schofield chipped in with, 'We're going to give you a makeover!'

Oh, God. Not a makeover. Anything but a TV make-over. They're not going to give me a makeover, are they?

I was in a pretty bad way cosmetically speaking; my skin was awful, I had spots and blemishes and had my fringe down over my forehead to hide this, as well as the necessary makeup. I couldn't have imagined anything worse than Phillip's shock revelation. I mean, I'd achieved the goal, I'd got my weight right down, I'd proved myself, but there was still a way to go and I wanted to get to that point before even entertaining the idea of being 'made over'. I know losing twenty stones was cause for celebration, but my personal goal was to lose another ten; twenty was just a good milestone on the way.

Then Lucy was brought out and it started getting a

bit like *This is your Life*. I started having flashbacks to me with Mum's hairbrush all those years ago. It could have got a bit embarrassing and overbearing for me, I think. But hey, it was a good time, it was a happy time and it was OK to milk it for all it was worth because it was unlikely that anything like this would ever happen again.

After the show we all went out and went on the London Eye and had lunch and champagne, but I didn't really touch much of it. The downer was kicking in again. I was talking to, looking at people I'd bonded with over the course of a year, knowing it had reached its conclusion and knowing I'd probably never see or hear from them ever again. It was difficult not to get upset. I was dealing with a lot in my personal life during the weight loss and maybe that was another factor to make me feel low. When I'd been as big as I was, I was actually considered to be disabled. I was given a monthly disability allowance from Social Services as well as support from them for things like cleaning the house as I just couldn't physically do it, as you know.

The money that I got from them was gratefully received because, as a junkie feeding my habit, I'd got myself into financial difficulty too. What with the taxis everywhere and the amount I was spending on food, I was living beyond my means and getting by on credit cards, overdrafts and loans and even remortgaging the house. This had all been going on for some time and was completely out of control. My wages didn't really cover all of my outgoings at all.

Once I was on my weight loss plan and got down to around thirty stones, I contacted Social Services to tell them I wanted to terminate my disability allowance. They were quite stunned because no one had ever contacted them to do this before. Maybe it was a bad move on my part, but I didn't feel disabled anymore and felt a bit guilty that I was getting fitter and felt the money would be of use to someone else. They told me that there were people who weighed less than me who were still eligible and were given disability allowance, so I was well within my rights to continue. I don't know; it would have got to the point where I'd feel I was cheating the system and I didn't want that at all. Losing that extra money did put me in a worse situation financially, but this had been money that I'd squander on junk food. I didn't need it. If I could still receive money for being in such a bad physical condition, that money was essentially keeping me there.

The next thing to take over from buying food was buying clothes. I couldn't help myself. It was the same thrill of finding something new. I'd never had proper clothes for years, and as I started to lose weight, clothes would actually fit me for once. But I bought clothes throughout the weight loss process and consequently owned every size of clothing you can imagine by the time I hit my target. I could have opened a clothes shop if I'd wanted. People were urging me not to keep buying, and I knew I shouldn't. It was just one of those things.

Clothes are such a great way of treating and rewarding yourself, and I was no different. I started to feel good about myself for the first time in God knows how long and there was no way I was going to wear my jogging pants and sweatshirts forever.

Back home from London, I did something I'd never done before: I sat there for three days without eating a thing. I'd never known what it was like to not have an appetite. It was literally from feeling deflated. The process was over, I'd kept my promise and gone on the show, it was a success, I didn't mess up ... and then there was a void, which would usually have been crammed full of food. It seemed there were too many comedowns in quick succession: the filming, the actual twenty stones journey, the screenings, the live appearance, the goodbye party ... And then nothing.

Until a 'media frenzy' ensued.

Just as I was preparing for normality, I was invited on to a chat show with Dr Chris in Ireland and then I was invited back on to *This Morning* to do a kind of presenting role soon after.

The show in Ireland was the Gerry Kelly show and to get there I went on a plane for the first time in my life! Being the size I was all those years, I'd never even chanced the embarrassment – there was no way I'd have been able to fit into one of the seats. Can you imagine the look of fear on people's faces if I turned up, weighing forty-four stones, to get on a plane? They'd have to counterbalance it by shoving more people on the other side so the plane didn't go round in circles. Dr Chris and I went along to Manchester Airport and I was amazed at how small the plane was. It wasn't one of your typical holiday-style planes and the flight was only around forty-five minutes. This was one of those flights that people made very regularly. For me, never having been on one before, regular flight was quite a lot to comprehend and the show just flying me over showed me how even air travel can be taken for granted. Boarding a plane was another achievement to add to the list! Me on a plane was bordering on the ridiculous. Oh, yes, and of course *This Morning* sent a camera crew up to catch it all on film ... as if I wasn't nervous enough. It was that odd mixture of excitement and fear, but I just had to get on with it. I had a camera with me to film the journey and got plenty of shots of Dr Chris giving the thumbs up sign. And then there was a camera crew waiting for us at the other side to film us touching down. In a way, it presented a false reality of what I was going through, because I couldn't back away from the plane screaming and have to be sedated like BA from *The A-Team*. Still, it was enjoyable and great that I had my friend with me.

To go on the show, I was nervous about having makeup on, because my skin complexion was quite bad at the time. And then there was the show itself. The only one I was used to at that point was *This Morning* and they were always supportive. I wasn't sure what to expect at all, and then found out that there would be a studio audience too. It's quite normal to be nervous before you do television, though, isn't it? I'm sure I can be excused. Gerry was a really nice bloke, we did the interview, I enjoyed it, it wasn't stressful, the audience was great ... no problems whatsoever. Dr Chris was there with me and we were also asked about how we'd become good friends as well as all the usual background questions about losing the weight. It seemed to be all over in seconds – a blur.

In the green room afterwards we met up with some of Dr Chris's relatives and Nancy Sorrell, wife of Vic Reeves, was also a guest on the show. I know she fancied me, but she's not my type. After that Dr Chris, his cousin Eamonn and his wife and I went for a lovely meal before heading back to the hotel that the *Gerry Kelly Show* had put us up in ... Officially the most bombed hotel in Europe.

Soon after touching down back at home, I was on *This Morning* again, talking about the healthy foods I ate. There was a chef making a healthy chilli, with me asking him all kinds of questions about it. They gave me a camera again and I was told to make the chilli at home to show how easy it could be. Doing things like this was something I'd soon get used to. I know I keep referring to my past life in times like this, but actually going on a TV show to discuss healthy food and talk about the healthy food I eat was madder than mad. If the Ghost of Christmas Future had visited me on that Christmas night in 2003 and showed me the scene in the studio of me, twenty-odd stone lighter and talking about being healthy, I don't think I'd have believed him. My entire life had been spent being unhealthy; to be asked on to a TV show as a credible 'expert' was ... well, *in*credible, a million miles from being Charlie Walduck.

Around a month later I was back doing a piece about curry and they kept asking me back when they wanted to do anything about healthy eating. Each time they'd always show a brief introduction of what I'd been up to since last being on the show and it was really nice to have such interest in me, in what I was doing and how I was living. I was on that many times I thought they were lining me up to take Phillip's job. It may have cost them a few quid less, but I'd have been up for it, no problem. Other than broadcast TV, there were so many newspaper articles and magazine features going on all the time. Literally, there have been hundreds of them from the build-up to going on *This Morning*, to doing the 10k and the marathon, to doing my own raising awareness initiatives, to doing anything, really. Sometimes it feels like it's just an excuse to feature me somewhere. Not that I'm complaining – any time I'm featured in a newspaper, there is a chance that at least one other person with obesity problems will be affected, so it has been worthwhile. Every time my story has been covered in a newspaper it has always been in a positive light and to promote good health, so I'm very pleased that I'm able to help in some way.

I did the Manchester 10k and the London Marathon in 2005. In my training for all this I ran with Mark, having actually kept our word and stayed in touch. We were going out on Thursday nights and doing 10k each time, running for short bursts and walking most of the time. When we started, I knew I didn't want to push myself too far and end up doing myself in. I told Mark it would be great to train with him, but I was going to walk the 10k rather than run. I said I'd run every now and then, but my goal was to complete it and, by walking, I knew it would be possible.

I was still a big lad then and probably a bit over twenty stone, and it was great to have the company. I was still really at the stage where I needed moral support. I know in describing my weight loss it sounds as though I suddenly became the most confident and fittest man alive, but that wasn't the case. I was still getting used to being able to move, and not exercising at all over those years had made me completely unfit. You need to train to get fit and I'd probably never fully be that until I shifted some more weight. A training partner really boosts your confidence and makes it less monotonous. One evening we were out walking and we turned a corner into one of my biggest fears. In front of us was a group of lads and I slowed right down. I said to Mark there was no way I could walk past them, never mind run past them. He told me to go for it – just keep my eyes forward, avoid any contact and we'd just head straight past. I hated this situation because I'd been in it so many times. We carried on and sure enough, as we neared them, one of them shouted.

'Oi!'

Eyes forward, take no notice.

'You're him off the telly who lost all that weight, aren't ya?'

Don't look, just keep walking.

'Well done, mate,' he said as we passed.

And they all gave us a huge round of applause as we went. It was amazing; a gang of stereotypical hoodies doing such a thing. Mark and I looked at each other as they were applauding and I was beaming from ear to ear. We both were.

And I walked past so many old dears who'd shout things like 'Charlie, get your knees up!' It was great to hear it and really gave me a boost each time it happened. It wasn't quite like Rocky running through the market, being thrown a piece of fruit and having a load of kids running with me up the escalators at the Trafford Centre, but you have to start somewhere, eh?

Once I was walking, there was no stopping me. I'd walk everywhere, determined to keep shedding the pounds. I couldn't believe that others weren't walking everywhere too. At work, instead of walking to the nearest shops with Beryl during our break, I wanted to go to the ones the furthest away. I must have been really doing her head in.

The Man on the Street: Top Five Insults

Or the woman on the street, or Joe Public, or the voice of the people, or a group of kids, or a couple of blokes, or a drunk ... whatever guise they wear, they all have the same mission. These are all people in life who take pleasure in being nasty to you either out of spite or just because they are too stupid to realise they are doing it. Sorry to sound slightly bitter here, but these people need to realise the effect their outbursts can have. I've had to put up with comments from these types all my life. They are disgusting, vile people.

Here are some of the confrontations I've had to endure over the years:

Straight in at number five: *I'll never win, so that makes me a what?* by A Gambler who Stunk of Cigarettes.

When some bloke stepped out of the betting shop in Failsworth and shouted, 'Put some weight on, have you?' I was livid. I replied to him by shouting two words in his direction. The first began with f and the second one was 'off'.

I hate to admit that I reacted by lowering myself to his level, but this was the only language he was likely to understand. And of course, he looked offended by my reaction, like I'd shouted at him for no reason.

'I was only joking,' he said.

'Only joking? Is anyone laughing?'

And he tutted and walked away. I hate confrontation, especially with people like him, because, more often than not, they generally didn't have the brains to discuss anything and would resort to violence within seconds. What a loser. I wonder how funny he'd have found it if I'd shouted 'Gambling addiction?' when he stepped out. This came when I was on track and losing weight. I'd gotten sick of people like him thinking they could shout abuse at me. I hadn't come so far just to get beaten by some moron. I had enough fight in me to stand up for myself and if that meant getting into a confrontation, then so be it. I knew I wouldn't get walked over again. They have no right to abuse anyone for living their life or try to make them feel bad about themselves.

At number four: *The grinning idiot* by A Grinning Idiot.

I was out in Manchester one day, and this was when I was quite big. I wasn't the biggest I've been, but big nonetheless, maybe thirty-five stone. As I walked past a bloke, he shouted, 'Oi, you!'

I turned to face him and he stepped towards me. I could tell that he wasn't out to make friends; he had a nasty look of spite in his whole demeanour.

'Excuse me. Do you mind if I ask you a question?' he asked.

Here we go again, I thought. *Witty and aggressive street philosophy by any chance?*

'Go on then. Ask me,' I sighed.

'How fat are you?' A smug look spread across his face like he'd just won his childish little game.

I took a deep breath. It was quite a predictable quip and, while he thought he was oh so hilarious, it just made him the most boring person in put-down history.

'Can I ask you a question then?' I replied. 'How big is your dick?'

This threw him right off guard and I could almost hear his tiny mind searching for a retort.

'Eleven and a half inches,' was his comeback.

'Well, I'm eleven and a half stone then,' was mine.

I walked away from him glad that I hadn't just kept my mouth shut.

Still at number three: *Aren't we really clever (no, really, aren't we)?* by A Bunch of Clever Football Fans

There were so many occasions at football matches where I experienced the wrath of 'the man on the street', the expert and social commentator that is the big-mouthed football idiot. I know it's a generalisation, but most of the negativity that I ever suffered through cruel jibes was at the hands of bully-boy terrace meatheads. At the same time, it was always quite a tribal thing. Being a Barrow fan meant that Barrow fans wouldn't abuse me. There'd be the ones who would in any other situation, but at a match, they knew they couldn't break the rules because I was one of them. Most people couldn't see that I was one of them anyway, no matter where we were in the world – a human being with feelings.

One incident was Barrow vs. Woking away. Fans weren't segregated then and you could go wherever you liked once in the ground, so after spotting the Barrow fans (it was sometimes difficult) I headed over in their direction. To get there, I had to walk past a stand filled with around a hundred, maybe more, Woking fans who saw me and decided to shout 'You fat bastard!' over and over. It used to get me angry that any human could treat another in such a way. It was so humiliating. They were never going to stop until I passed them and being right in front and having so many people project such hate in my direction was soul destroying. I was crying inside and couldn't let it show on the outside. I just had to struggle past. It was pointless reacting, pointless pretending I hadn't heard them.

I'd paid money to travel down and for a ticket to watch my team just to be abused by such horrible excuses for men, stood there in the safety of their pack thinking they had the right to call someone and make him feel bad about himself.

I felt so helpless, being such a long way from home and having that happen to me. If it had been a home game, I'd probably have just left. I had the whole match and the travelling back to let it eat away at me, but I did get the last laugh as we won 3–2. A big 'well done' to those brave men for picking on another who was a bit different from them, one that was obviously struggling with his weight, and then to initiate a chorus like that, singling him out even more and punishing him further, making him feel the worst he could in front of hundreds of people – you can be proud of yourselves. Mission accomplished. It was a shame to go to Paul Weller's home town of all places to endure such behaviour. Why do we treat each other like that?

10 DOWNING STREET
LONDON SW1A 2AA
www.pm.gov.uk

THE PRIME MINISTER

23 October 2006

Dear Charlie,

Thanks for sending a copy of your open letter to me in the Evening Mail.

It was very good timing because it arrived in my office on the very day that the Government announced our plans to give better personal support and encouragement to people to live healthier lives.

You are right to say that Governments can't make the public eat healthily or take exercise. But we can work harder to give people the support to make the right choices themselves. And the more we can personalise that help and deliver it locally, the better that will be.

So that's exactly what we are going to do. We are linking up with local supermarkets, with chemists, fitness trainers, gyms and councils to see what we can together do to give people the support they need to lose weight, keep fit, quit smoking and lead healthier lifestyles.

Although I can't promise we have taken on board all your ideas, I hope you will find that we are thinking on the same lines.

- 2 -

In fact, some of your ideas such as healthy living centres, fitness trainers on prescription, better school meals and improved food labelling are already being put into practice either locally or across the whole country.

Have a look at the *Health Challenge England* report setting out the sort of things we want to encourage. Congratulations on all you have achieved.

Yours sincerely,

Tony Blair

Mr Charlie Walduck

A nice letter from Tony.

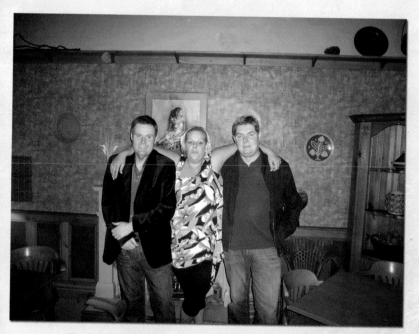

Me with Jackie and Steven after I'd slimmed down a bit.

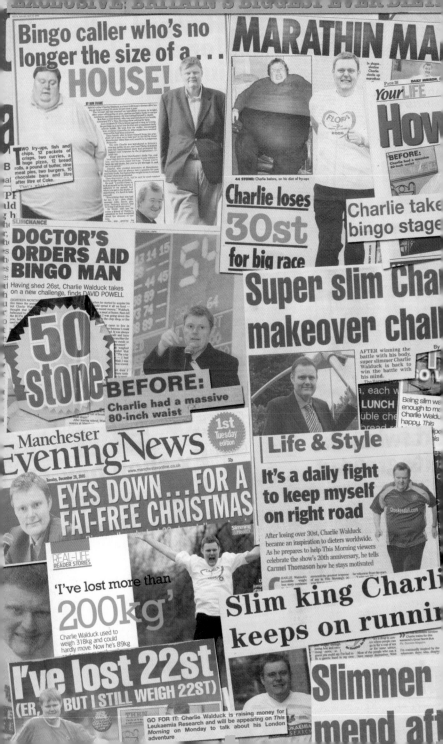

Bingo caller who's no longer the size of a . . . HOUSE!

MARATHIN MA

Your LIFE

How

BEFORE: Charlie had a massive 80-inch waist

44 STONE: Charlie before, on his diet of fry-ups

Charlie loses 30st for big race

Charlie take bingo stage

DOCTOR'S ORDERS AID BINGO MAN

Having shed 26st, Charlie Walduck takes on a new challenge, finds DAVID POWELL

Super slim Cha makeover chall

50 stone

BEFORE: Charlie had a massive 80-inch waist

AFTER winning the battle with his body, super slimmer Charlie Walduck is back to win the battle with his mind.

LUNCH

Being slim we enough to ma Charlie Waldu happy. This

Manchester Evening News

1st Tuesday edition

Tuesday, December 20, 2005   www.manchesteronline.co.uk

EYES DOWN . . . FOR A FAT-FREE CHRISTMAS

Life & Style

It's a daily fight to keep myself on right road

After losing over 30st, Charlie Walduck became an inspiration to dieters worldwide. As he prepares to help This Morning viewers celebrate the show's 20th anniversary, he tells Carmel Thomason how he stays motivated

REAL-LIFE READER STORIES

'I've lost more than 200kg'

Charlie Walduck used to weigh 318kg and could hardly move. Now he's 89kg

Slim king Charli keeps on runnin

I've lost 22st (ER, BUT I STILL WEIGH 22ST)

GO FOR IT: Charlie Walduck is raising money for Leukaemia Research and will be appearing on This Morning on Monday to talk about his London adventure

Slimmer mend af

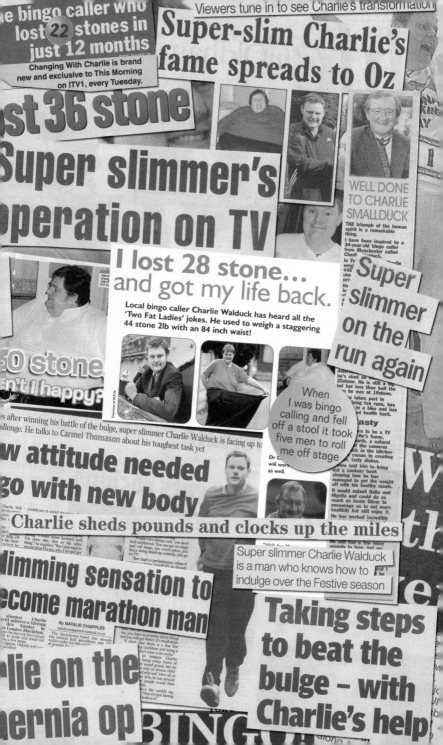

e bingo caller who lost 22 stones in just 12 months

Changing With Charlie is brand new and exclusive to This Morning on ITV1, every Tuesday.

Viewers tune in to see Charlie's transformation

Super-slim Charlie's fame spreads to Oz

st 36 stone

Super slimmer's peration on TV

WELL DONE TO CHARLIE SMALLDUCK

THE triumph of the human spirit is a remarkable thing.

I have been inspired by a 34-year-old bingo caller from Manchester called Charlie...duck.

Super slimmer on the run again

I lost 28 stone... and got my life back.

Local bingo caller Charlie Walduck has heard all the 'Two Fat Ladies' jokes. He used to weigh a staggering 44 stone 2lb with an 84 inch waist!

When I was bingo calling and fell off a stool it took five men to roll me off stage

0 stone n't I happy?

s after winning his battle of the bulge, super slimmer Charlie Walduck is facing up to allenge. He talks to **Carmel Thomason** about his toughest task yet

w attitude needed o with new body

Charlie sheds pounds and clocks up the miles

Super slimmer Charlie Walduck is a man who knows how to indulge over the Festive season

imming sensation to ecome marathon man

By NATALIE CHAPPLES

natalie.chapples@nwnail.co.uk

Taking steps to beat the bulge – with Charlie's help

lie on the ernia op

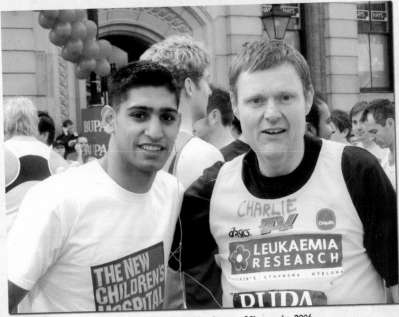

With Amir Khan at the BUPA Manchester 10k run in 2006.

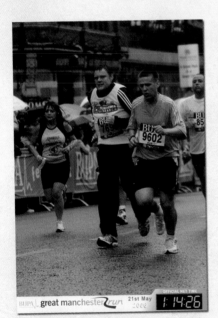

On the run ... Thanks to Nicola for looking after me and treating me like a real celebrity.

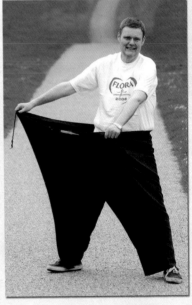

Me with my big pants before the London Marathon (they were hard to run in).

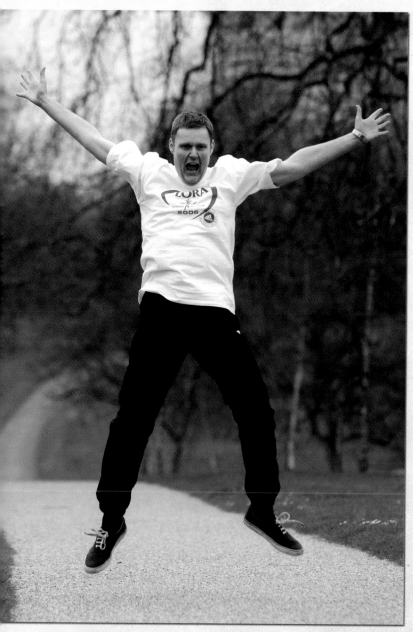

Jumping for joy in Hyde Park before the London Marathon in 2006

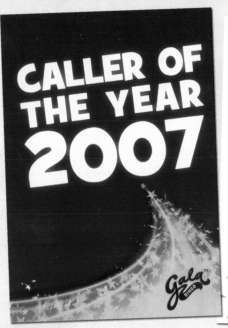

CALLER OF THE YEAR 2007

REGION 6:
Charles Walduck
(Belle Vue)

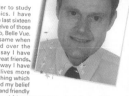

I am thirty eight years old, live in Failsworth, Manchester. Originally from Barrow-in-Furness in Cumbria, I moved to Manchester to study a degree in Economics. I have worked in bingo for the last sixteen years, having spent twelve of those years at my current club, Belle Vue. No two days are the same when working in bingo and over the years I am proud to say I have met and made many great friends. I hope in some small way I have made our customers lives more fulfilled – that is something which I always strive to do and my belief is that to some, a smile and friendly greeting can make the difference between a good or a bad day. Knowing that makes me feel good too.

During my time at Gala bingo I have had many highlights and it is always nice to see people win big. I am also proud to have helped raise thousands of pounds for charity over the years as well as helping to establish the club as a real hub of the community.

To win the title of **GALA CALLER OF THE YEAR 2007** would be wonderful achievement for me. To be judged as the best in my profession would mean more to me than anything else.

Charles

I won through to the Gala Bingo Caller of the Year final in 2007.
I didn't win, but two weeks later I was off to Oz, so I didn't really care.

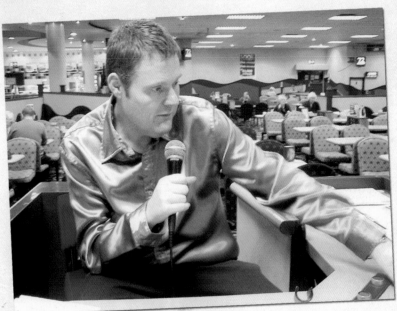

Calling at Belle Vue in my gold shirt (stylish or what?).

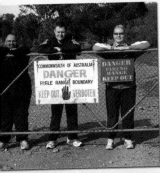

Mick and his wife Linda in happier times [wei]ght loss camp in Australia).

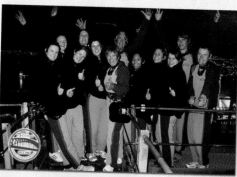

Me on top of the Sydney Harbour Bridge.

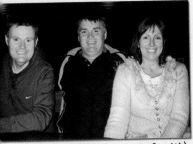

(who I did the Mudgee fun run in Oz with) [and] his girlfriend Carolyn.
[Gla]d that they both found love with each other.

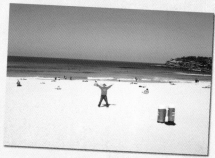

Me on Bondi Beach.
Always wished I had the body for it.

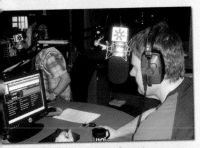

[Wor]king on the radio, in my element.

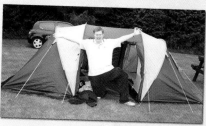

Camping with Lucy in 2006.

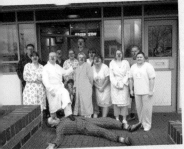

[P]romoting Red Nose Day outside the bingo hall [w]ith all my bingo pals. I'm the one on the floor.

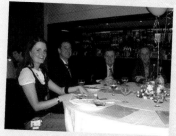

On a charity night with Mark to the left of me. I am proud to say that I've raised almost £15,000 for charity doing my runs and walks.

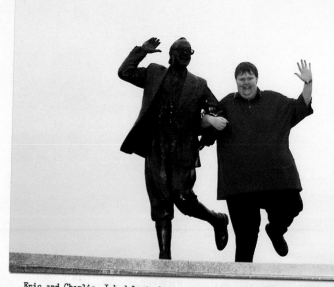

Eric and Charlie. I had lost about sixteen stones at this point (November 2004) ...

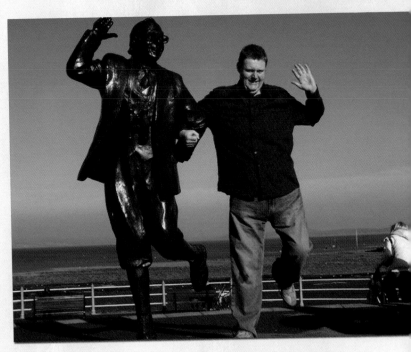

... and then about twenty-eight stones at this point a year later.

Why do we take pleasure in hurting people so much? If they knew the agony I was in just walking past them, the agony of sitting for such a long journey, the agony of standing ... would they still have done it? I'd hate to know the real answer.

Up two places to number two: *I've run out of anything to say, you got me back and now I want to fight you* by A Football Yob

Once I got off the train at Bolton for a match and there were two blokes wearing Bolton shirts walking towards me. They saw me and obviously said something to each other with a laugh and a nudge as we got closer. I was so tired of seeing this look on other people's faces. It wasn't worth just turning and walking away because there wasn't much I hadn't heard. It was like that *Father Ted* scene where Ted gets the idea of saying 'I don't believe it!' to Richard Wilson. It was always a million miles from being funny.

And then it came with such venom.

'You fat bastard,' one of them said.

He was right in my face, aggressive. It was the equivalent of just walking up to me and punching me – that was the kind of damage he was looking to cause.

'I'd rather be a fat bastard than a Bolton fan,' I replied.

They stopped in their tracks and he was dumb(struck). 'What did you say?'

I told him again, and he actually went for me! His mate was pulling him back and I told him something to the effect of 'Don't give it if you can't take it.'

People like him disgust me. I could have lowered myself to his level and verbally attacked him if I'd wanted, but it seemed I hit a raw nerve by insulting

177

his beloved football team instead. I've got nothing against Bolton anyway; it was just the first thing that sprung to mind because of his shirt. He wasn't the best-looking bloke in the world; I could have called him ugly bastard, he had a big nose ... big-nosed bastard, he was short ... little bastard ... he had no hair ... baldy bastard ... I could go on. He could have had any prefix, really.

And still at number one: *I'm too daft to know fruit is good for you, but I'll try to put you down in public anyway* by A N Oying Woman

Once I was eating an apple in the street and a woman approached me and said, 'Are you allowed to eat that?'

I was stunned. I looked at the apple and then at her.

'Are you allowed to eat one?' I asked.

'Yes,' she said.

'Well ... you're fatter than me, love. So, yes. I am allowed to eat it,' and off I walked.

I had to pinch myself to make sure it wasn't a dream. And then she looked at me as if I'd been the one having a go. I wasn't meaning to be rude to her, but what was she expecting coming out with something like that to someone she doesn't even know?

As long as there are people, there will be insults. I'm not the type to comment on anyone's appearance, it's a horrible thing to do. The smallest comment can have a massive effect on a person's state of mind. It is magnified if it comes from a friend or family member because it's more personal.

When it came to the day of the Manchester 10k, the organisers were brilliant. They knew I'd be walking it and they still put me in pole position up there at the front with the elite runners and the celebrities. These were some of the fastest runners in the world and it was slightly daunting. With *This Morning* being part of it all, they had me chaperoned by Julie Dawn Cole for the run. Julie is the show's fitness expert and was only Veruca Salt in the original *Willy Wonka and the Chocolate Factory* film. How cool is that? I didn't even know she'd been in the film when we met, but if I had I wouldn't have talked about anything else, because I *love* that film. God knows what the elite runners were thinking when they saw us alongside them. When we started, I was literally dragged along with them, unable to stop but unable to run too. I was walking within a few seconds and was sure it was Christopher Eccleston who'd pushed me along – pesky ex-time lord! · I did run bits of it – it was impossible not to because of the cheering and how good it made me feel – and finished the 10k in one hour and fifty minutes. It wasn't a bad effort at all.

As I crossed the finish line, *This Morning* had a

camera crew there to capture the moment, which put the BBC's nose out of place a bit because they wanted to interview me first. I met a load of ace people that day: Liz Dawn from *Coronation Street* and Sue Johnston from *The Royle Family* (and *Face* by Antonia Bird) were there at the start, Tony Audenshaw and Chris Chittell (Bob Hope and Eric Pollard) from *Emmerdale* and, of course, the doctor from *Doctor Who* (he's not a real doctor). The best bit about it was, well ... was all of it. Any time something like this was on TV in the past, I would never have stayed on the channel for more than a couple of seconds. Running was just alien to me; there was no point in watching as it would just upset me. But then there was the new-and-improved me actually taking part, completing it and being interviewed after it!

Seeing the crew from *This Morning* at the end made it special because it almost gave a real ending to the weight loss process, from joking around and saying I'd do it on that first day of meeting them to actually losing all the weight and staying true to my word. I know it's their job to be professional, but with the time we all spent together, the support they offered and the friendship that evolved, I know they were as chuffed as I was when I stepped over the finishing line.

Steve the producer had been in touch with me throughout the filming by text message, phone calls and e-mails and it was that kind of dedication that kept *me* dedicated. Likewise with Dr Chris; if he hadn't been in regular contact, if he was someone who didn't care as much as he did and want me to succeed, I wouldn't have. Everyone who was part of the crew, part of *This Morning* was behind me and I'm so grateful for all they did.

I've now done the run every year since, other than

when I was away in Australia, getting my time down to one hour twenty-five in 2009. The organisers asked me to put my name to a fitness initiative to encourage more people to take to the streets and get mobile, which I did, and I helped to promote it alongside boxers Amir Khan and Ricky Hatton, Paralympic gold medallist Tanni Grey-Thompson, Kelly Holmes and Tony Audenshaw, and we all had to run the first mile of the 10k. There were two youngsters with us who'd won the kids' run the previous day. I think I was as excited as the kids were. It was such an honour for me to get the recognition and be thought of as someone who'd give the campaign further credibility. I loved being part of things like that.

The day after the 10k I was on the show talking about my achievement and told the nation I was going to do the Great North Run next. Lorraine Kelly was co-hosting. 'No! It's all uphill, that!' she said.

It isn't strictly all uphill, but I know what she meant. I'd set my sights on it by then and there wasn't much that could stop me. I suppose it was part 'I told you I could do it' and part 'Wow. I *can* do it' that was spurring me on. I also used my training for these runs and walks as further exercise to lose that bit more weight. It was a win–win situation.

Mark and I even stepped up the pace a bit. The walking got to the point where I could actually jog, not just walking quickly and jogging for a few steps, actual jogging! The lead-up to the run was a bit hectic because the day before was Charlie's Hearty Walk, which kicked off at Manchester City's ground, filmed by Granada for a TV advert, and I was also interviewed on the ITN lunchtime news. The photo shoot for this one saw me surrounded by three busty blonde glamour models, who were amazing to work with, and again, and unfortunately for them, they just weren't my type.

The Great North Run is a half marathon and one of the most famous in the world. There I was, Charlie the bingo caller from Failsworth, rubbing shoulders with the fastest runners on the planet – again – and some household celebrity names. I was put up in the posh Copthorne Hotel in Newcastle the night before (totally looked after as one expects) and was up bright and early for the run the following morning, escorted to the starting line by our chaperone, Richard, who ran along with us. You find with the celebrity runners that there are always the same ones doing charity runs. They are either the keen athletic ones like Nell McAndrew or the ones who aren't that well known for their fitness, but who've trained their heart out to do the run and raise money and awareness for a cause. Good on them. And the BBC got their interview this time as part of the Great North Run programme.

Justine from *This Morning* arranged for me to see a top surgeon who 'does' all the celebrities in London. It was filmed for the show. He said he didn't really want to do the job because it was too big. The job was to remove all the loose skin on my body. As you'll probably know, being so fat had stretched my skin to its limit and losing that amount of weight meant there was so much excess skin left on me. He felt that I wouldn't look 100 per cent after doing what he could and, as his job was all about giving people confidence and perfection, he didn't think it was possible to achieve it. *Fairy nuff*, I thought. Had it been a few tucks here and there, then maybe he'd have done it.

I asked my doctor about it and went for tests, as-sessments, photographs, on a waiting list, tests, assessments, appointments, another waiting list ... and then a date came in for me to have surgery on the NHS. Going through all the tests was quite difficult because, in a way, you almost have to play the system to your own advantage. For example, if you go in there and tell them you desperately need surgery because it will change your life forever, then your expectations are too high and they won't authorise surgery. And on the other hand, if you go in saying that you aren't that bothered, you are talking your way out of surgery. So, I had to say I needed surgery in order to go for a wee properly and to get jeans that would fit without this massive overhang. They told me it wouldn't change my life completely and I said I knew that, as long as it helped in those areas mentioned, then I'd be happier in myself.

It wasn't a huge operation, just a bit of the loose skin removed around my stomach, which totalled around ten pounds. Annoyingly, with it being on TV and in newspapers, the bit that stuck in people's minds was that I'd had surgery. And putting two and two together, it was assumed that this was weight loss surgery, rather than what it really was.

I was approached by someone in the street (as I am) who commented that I'd lost weight, and then he said, 'Because you had surgery, didn't you?' and walked off while I was telling him what the surgery was. It was a disappointment because it took away the credibility that I'd done it all by myself. One tiny tuck and it was assumed I'd had thirty stone vacuumed out. The surgery itself was really helpful though. The skin I had removed was below my stomach, I suppose where a bloke's beer belly would be, as it had presented a few difficulties when going to the toilet. I was in hospital for five days and it healed up really well.

After becoming Runner Charlie, it was time to be Traveller Charlie for a bit. I'd always set myself goals when I was losing weight and it was time to fulfil them properly by booking myself on a flight to Canada. The time I flew to Ireland with Dr Chris had been my first, but I needed to experience it properly on a long flight in a proper big plane to actually say I'd done it. The other flight had been an exciting experience, but I'd had meals that had lasted longer and Canada certainly wouldn't be a blink-and-miss-it flight. It would be packed with passengers going on holiday rather than a toy flight across the Irish Sea.

It was just like walking really. Once I could walk I wanted to do it more and go further and it was the same with travelling. Not that I turned into Alan Whicker overnight, but just to do something I'd never had the chance to do, being up in the air as a normal passenger, was achieving something else I'd longed for. For me to even set foot on a plane in the past would have put me on the bill of the in-flight entertainment for all the wrong reasons. I'd have been the butt of all the cruel jibes and one of the stories the holidaymakers would recall to friends and family on their return. And I'd have felt a burden because there'd have been consequences of sitting for too long with my comfort and circulation, assuming I could sit in the first place.

So Canada it was. For a day. I knew they'd speak English in Toronto and that was what I wanted. I flew out on a Monday, spent Tuesday there and was back in Manchester on the Wednesday! All I took was an overnight bag; everyone at the airport was baffled.

'How long are you staying in Canada, sir?'

'Just a night, thanks.'

I don't know if I was offending them, come to think about it. I stayed in a hotel that I'd booked separately from the flight, and of course it turned out to be situated in a rather rough suburb of Toronto. The room wasn't up to much and I got in, sat on the bed, switched the TV on and wondered what the hell I was doing there. You know when you get somewhere and there just aren't the home comforts you're used to and it's a bit of a letdown? It was a bit of a 'We've gone on holiday by mistake' *Withnail* moment, but at least I'd only booked to stay there for a night. I went out for a walk, forgetting that cars drive on the other side, and was nearly roadkill within five minutes. When I recovered, I walked to a bus station so I could suss out how to get to the city centre the next day.

I was quite the tourist, doing the CN Tower, going on a sightseeing bus trip and didn't go to Niagara Falls, which I wish I had done now. On my way back to the hotel on the bus, I noticed a bingo hall, so when I got back and freshened up, I had a walk up there for a couple of games.

As soon as I was home, my focus was on the London Marathon for April the following year. Mark and I were back in Thursday training. My flight landed in the early hours of Thursday morning, so we kept our regular Thursday evening date. Mark knew by doing the runs with me that he was helping me to keep the weight off. He'd helped me try to lose weight in the past and, knowing that he hadn't been part of the big journey, he still said he'd help me out in whatever way he could.

In December that year I reached my weight loss target and got down to fourteen stone, meaning I had lost thirty stones in twenty months. Give or take the odd pound, my mission was complete. This was the real journey for me. This was the one I'd always set my sights on, although I missed the camera crews and everything that went with it because they'd been with me literally from day one. To reach my goal alone was the right way to do it though. It was a personal journey after all and I'd got to where I wanted to be. I had such a sense of achievement and still do when I think about it. I'd gone from, let's face it, the brink of death to getting down to a size that is associated with 'normal living'.

I was in touch with Dr Chris throughout this, still meeting up with him for walks and chats and picking his brains on a few things. I hit a low ebb soon after this, despite the fact that I was doing so much more with my life. As I said earlier, I believe those thoughts, feelings, emotions, depression, and dark, desperate times will always be there, I just needed to have coping strategies in place. I don't know what was fuelling this particular bout because life was good at the time and it just shows that it can hit you however well you are doing. I think that my defences were down from the whole process coming to an end, regular social contact with those from the show and the film crew was over and the routine of it all was gone, never to come back. I'd always look at it in a negative way, rather than a positive. And of course, there was the financial aftermath of a lifetime of eating to deal with. So, although my life was getting back on track and I was able to start living like everyone else, it seemed I had to pick up the pieces from my former life and there was still much to resolve.

Dr Chris always knew the right words: 'Charlie, if you ever feel low, just keep thinking of what you have achieved and the encouragement and help you must have given to thousands of people with weight problems. You have been an inspiration and a great example of what can be achieved once you put your mind to it. Your story has been one of great personal motivation, self-discipline and success. Sorry to go on, but I really am so very proud of you, and you should also feel proud of what you have achieved – well done!'

I was back on *This Morning* at Christmas doing Charlie's Choices and was so involved with the show that I bet Phillip was secretly worried. I did Charlie's Choices a few times on the show. It was all about low-fat ready meals, what to look for, what to look out for, that kind of thing. The Christmas one was looking at cutting down on fatty foods over the season, what not to snack on, differences in cooking oils, and even discussed not having gravy on Christmas dinner and cutting down on alcohol because it leads to snacking when you get a false hunger. Controversial or what? It's nice to get asked back regularly; it's like visiting friends every few months. It always gave me a lift and kept the connection. To say that being on the show has transformed my life is a slight understatement. If I'd known the positive effect of Lucy writing that letter, I'd have told her to do it much earlier. No one could have predicted the results or the response. Since being on the show, I get recognised all the time and it is always in such a positive way that it makes me proud to be alive. The best thing about it is being able to help others. No matter how corny that sounds, I'm now in a position where people look to me for help, much in the same way I looked to Dr Chris.

I get e-mails and phone calls from people wanting advice or just wanting to say hello and wish me luck. It's that kind of contact that keeps me on the straight and narrow and reels me back in any time I might be straying from eating well. It sometimes makes me wonder about all those idiots on the street who used to shout abuse. Do they remember me? Did they watch the films? Did it affect them; did they learn something about me? And I suppose the irony is that I ended up skinnier than most of them anyway. I bet they felt a bit sick about that. Especially the Bolton fan.

By now, I should have been prepared for a big low to see the high off. And boy did it come in grand fashion. I had massive stomach pains towards the end of 2005 and went to the hospital, because I could feel a lump in my stomach. I was told it was a deposit of hard skin because of my weight loss, was given some antibiotics to last that day and was due to go back the following day for more. I was in too much pain. The next day I went to see my doctor. He told me to go home, lie down, not do anything and he was going to send an ambulance round immediately. It turned out that I had a strangulated hernia and went in to have an operation on New Year's Eve. What a way to see the New Year in! I was very lucky though because the hernia had turned gangrenous and I'd have been in a serious condition if I'd just taken antibiotics. It was caught just in time. So, the first year when I could go out and enjoy myself, I was stuck in hospital. I was asleep well before midnight, exhausted, and laid up for a good few days before, during and after. While I was in there, *This Morning* was back on TV and they wished me well and sent a bunch of flowers. It was nice of them and created a bit of a buzz in the ward. Of course, when the doctors came round to check that I was OK, they said they could have sorted out *all* my loose skin while they were on with my hernia. I was so tempted to tell them to knock me out there and then and do it.

I'm certainly not in any rush to have the loose skin removed now. I know these days that my weight does fluctuate and any weight that I do put on goes straight to where the loose skin is. In fairness, it would take a lot of surgery to put it right and I'd end up looking like a patchwork quilt for a good while. So, I've never been at a point where the time has been right or I've definitely wanted it done; I'm happy as I am for now.

I was conscious not to let being in hospital put me off my training for the London Marathon. This was one of those obstacles that could have escalated and become a life issue if I dwelled on it; the perfect excuse to stay indoors, the perfect excuse to revert to old ways, seek solace and fall off the wagon. I didn't let it happen. Once I was able to, Mark and I went back to our 10k training routine. He wasn't around to do the run itself, but still helped me train for it. Then in April 2006, just over two years since starting my weight loss plan, I completed the run in six hours and forty-five minutes. This was one of my greatest achievements ever; the biggest goal on my list. I mean, if you are driving or boarding a train or a plane to go somewhere and you're told it will take nearly seven hours to get there, you don't want to go. Then to do a trip of the same dura-tion, but having to run it – it's just mental. Doing a 10k and a thirteen-mile run were big enough achievements, but as Ray Winstone would probably tell me, doing a marathon is the daddy of all running achievements. Before, I couldn't have lived without eating for that length of time: now I could run it.

Again, I was put up in a nice hotel the night before, and the following day I made my way to the bus to get driven to the start line. I was in the same hotel as all the elite runners and was given a pass to board the same bus as them. Looking slightly out of place, I checked my pass and it read 'Charlie Walduck: Elite Runner'. It could have got embarrassing if any of them

189

questioned me, so I just kept schtum until we got to the start and joined the rest of the runners. I saw the group G4 (*XFactor*, 2004), Andrew Castle, Jade Goody and, of course, I was filmed by *This Morning* throughout.

I felt on top of the world after doing the marathon; it is one of those defining moments in my life. I was back on the show the day after the run, and this to me was where the real weight loss story ended. I pretty much knew I was the only one who remembered me even saying I'd do the London Marathon on that first day of filming. They all thought I was joking, but I wasn't. It was my overall goal – lose thirty stones and get fit enough to do the marathon. And there it was. Done.

In my capacity as Traveller Charlie, I took a five-week break in Australia soon after this. It was a bit of a mad adventure. I received an e-mail from a guy called Mick Organ inviting me to visit, having seen my story on YouTube. He wanted me to come out and inspire some of his clients at the Mudgee Weight Loss and Lifestyle Services in New South Wales.

It was a great opportunity, but could I do it? Could I meet a complete stranger and spend a whole month living with him and his family? Was this an opportunity too good to miss? Going to Australia had always been a dream of mine and it would tie in with my travelling goals, especially as it is the other side of the world. Everyone told me I should go for it and my head and my heart were on their side. Management at work were not as keen, though. Five weeks, maybe six if you add readjustment time, off work is quite a lot to ask of an employer, but not if they are an ex-employer. So I decided to quit my job. It wasn't an ultimatum or anything as dramatic, I just decided to make a massive change and take control of my own destiny. I waved goodbye to Manchester and said g'day to Australia.

I had a brilliant time there and am pleased to say

that I made some great and wonderful friends. I managed to help, encourage and support some people to lose weight too. It was bizarre; I was now considered to be a 'face' for change and turning an unhealthy life into a healthy one. And not just on my own doorstep. I didn't always see eye to eye with Mick's techniques. I think shouting at people to lose weight is the wrong approach, but it's horses for courses, isn't it? He may think that my technique of listening, understanding, relating and encouraging is too much of a softly-softly approach. But shouting does motivate people too. I just think you need the balance of someone who understands, like a good cop.

I have seen quite a few charlatans set up their own weight loss camps over the years and even got involved with one of them for a while. Dr Chris and I went along to this 'fat camp' until we realised the bloke who was running it was full of what he talked, if you get what I mean. It was terrible. OK, you don't need to be medically qualified to give advice, but you owe it to the people who are paying you to at least know some facts and be able to give them something tangible.

There are so many slimming clubs around now too. I knew a lady who lost thirty stones going to a slimming club: it was the same stone thirty times. This is the problem with most of the clubs; you go along lose weight, lose interest, put it back on and then go back and try again. I'm not knocking all of them, just like I wasn't knocking all gyms. They all work for some people, or they wouldn't be able to stay open.

The social aspect of going to a club can never be disputed and, if you can get the support you need to see you through, then it may just well work for you. Just bear in mind that some of them don't encourage exercise and are held in pretty miserable surroundings, and some don't offer an ongoing support network, which I think is vital.

My Auntie Doreen used to go to one and still might for all I know. They would all go to the chippy afterwards to celebrate their weight loss, safe in the knowledge that they had a whole week in which to lose those extra pounds again. It always used to make me laugh.

Other people wrote into the show asking for the same kind of help I received too. They saw my transformation, and being in a similar position, wanted *This Morning* and Dr Chris to save them. There was a woman called Sheila in Bath who wrote a letter and we went to see her and offered her all the support we could. I've helped anyone who has contacted me because I love being able to help others. I know exactly how these people feel and I did honestly feel that after going through it myself I knew many of the answers they'd be searching for.

I visited Sheila twice getting a coach down to see her, all out of my own pocket, and it seemed like a complete waste of time. It's not like a bus to Bath was just round the corner either, but I said I'd go to help out and see how she was getting on.

Her husband was the main problem in her life. He came out with such gems as 'Maybe you won't love me anymore if you lose weight.' He was a big guy himself and it never looked like there was commitment from him or her to achieve what she wanted. Her heart wasn't in it and he didn't appear to be supportive, so there wasn't really a goal. It was a complete waste of time and felt like she was just curious to see what might happen if she could be bothered, rather than wanting to change her life in any way.

I think because people saw me lose such a vast amount of weight over the course of five days on their TV they thought it was easy. Sheila probably wanted a quick fix. It was easy to get the impression that a miracle cure had occurred for me from watching it on the show, but we know it was a lot of hard graft over the course of many months. There wasn't a magic wand.

Being so busy while in Australia, sometimes I didn't get the opportunity to take a step back and realise the enormity of what I'd done. I had a bit of 'me time' during the visit and was able to appreciate my achievements. I'd come a long way. Literally. I appeared on Channel 9 TV as well as doing the Mudgee Fun Run, newspaper interviews and spent a lot of time with guys there who were on a weight loss programme. I was proud to be able to take a lad called Sam around on his first-ever fun run and it was such a great achievement for the guy. Being asked to go over there to help people was unreal and it was nice to do the run as I missed doing the Manchester 10k while there.

It was amazing getting recognised by people even in Australia. I was in a cafe in Melbourne and was approached by a woman who did the old 'It's Charlie from *This Morning*!' I was also recognised in Mudgee by an English woman. 'What are you doing here, Charlie?'

I also sampled a local delicacy. Kangaroo. I can't say I enjoyed it too much; I kept looking over my shoulder to see if Ant and Dec were going to give me a gold star. Kangaroo is low in fat with a very strong ... er ... kangarooey taste. I'm not that into rare meat either and this was so rare it was practically hopping off my plate. I like getting recognised, but at the same time, if

I'm recognised in somewhere like a cafe, they'll talk to me and be looking at my plate. And there are people out there who will comment, just like the ones I've mentioned within these pages. For every ten positive people congratulating me, there'll always be one negative: 'You can't have that, can you?'

Maybe I should have been conscious that I was out there practically in a different world but, in my own world I'd left behind, I was jobless. But I really wanted to take the opportunity to see as much as I could because it isn't every day you get to travel to a place like Australia. I have always been a big worrier too, so I thought if I was to plan and execute a massive trip it would either kill me or cure me of my fears. If I could go on such a journey, then I might not worry about little things in the future.

In 2008 I returned after another invite from Mick. It was a second chance-of-a-lifetime opportunity and this time I saw a lot more of the sights, going to Sydney, Adelaide, Perth, Melbourne, Tasmania, Darwin, Cairns and Brisbane on train, bus, ferry and plane. I even went snorkelling in the Great Barrier Reef. And when I got back home, there was an e-mail waiting for me from a man who thought he spotted me in Melbourne, but his wife insisted it couldn't have been me. They'd had an argument over it and he asked if I could put the record straight.

L osing thirty stones in twenty months is just nuts to even imagine. Dr Chris said that there hadn't been anything like it ever recorded in the UK to his knowledge, so it made me an unofficial record breaker. To go from being a fat bloke abused in the street to being known as a 'super slimmer' took a lot of dedication (and getting used to), but here's one thing I maintain and something you should always keep in mind too: losing weight isn't rocket science. At the most, it is simple mathematics and willpower. That's what it took – no special foods, no expensive supplements or pills and no expensive surgery.

The thing with doing this is that you don't have to fork out all the time. I did it without having to join a gym for hundreds of pounds a year and didn't have to drink a dozen protein shakes a day and allow myself a lettuce leaf and half a carrot for a special treat every other. Simplicity was the way forward.

You don't need a gym membership if you have streets and countryside when you open your front door. Once I'd lost weight, I went to a gym just to see what all the fuss was about. And, as most of you will know, there are different kinds of gyms. There's the typical old-school bloke's gym where you go to lift heavy weights – full of grunting and testosterone, spitting on the floor and chinning a punch bag. Then there are the WAGs in Lycra and poseurs gym where no one seems to do anything but look in the mirror. Last but not least, there are plenty of people-friendly ones that don't cost an arm and a leg. I'm not knocking gyms at all here. It's just that my needs were completely different from the needs of someone wanting to work out. You can try out any gym in the land before signing up and most of them will offer special deals, especially if you go in January when they are trying to encourage new members.

The one I went to wasn't top of the range and was accessible to all. I was amazed, though: people were still paying money to go on a walk or a run. Of course, there are other exercises to do, but I just couldn't get my head round it all. I didn't see the point in paying to go indoors on a running machine, especially when it was set to walking pace.

If you can formulate blinkered points of view like mine above rather than paying money you think you need to spend, then you'll be saving your hard-earned cash for more essential things.

There's one other snippet you always need to bear in mind if starting a diet, and this is the most important one: *If Charlie can do it, I can do it.*

Old wives' tales are very true too. I've never met one of these old wives; I don't know how old they are or who they're married to, but they must know everything. Remember the old saying 'You are what you eat'? Well, that was me. Pies, crisps, pizza, fry-ups, massive portions, late-night meals ... I was all of that. Fat. That was it. I didn't eat anything healthy and, as a result, I wasn't healthy. And eating lots of unhealthy foods made me extremely unhealthy. And guess what eating fat made me.

Here's my massive weight loss secret: all things in moderation. Another wives' tale, another simple concept and one that works. It's about energy in and energy out: consume less and exercise more. And here's how I didn't lose weight:

Atkins diet, just drinking water diet, hip and thigh diet, grape and melon diet, starving myself stupid diet, the watercress soup diet, the Madonna uses this one (I know because it was in *heat* magazine) diet, Beyoncé's diet, hypnosis, acupuncture, aversion therapy, aromatherapy, hydrotherapy, regression therapy, drugs (of any kind), protein drinks, fancy milkshakes, fancy cuppa soups, meal-replacement food bars, stomach bypass surgery, jaws wired up, locked in a dungeon.

There are so many diets out there that are just fads and may work to lose *some* weight. If you consume just watery stuff for a few weeks, you'll lose weight. If you don't eat, you'll also lose some weight. It stands to reason. Until you start eating again. Or you die of starvation.

The diets in most magazines serve as quick fixes and are marketed as 'bikini diets' for a reason. Don't do one of them if you want to sustain weight loss: they are just geared towards someone wanting to fit into their bather and look a bit slimmer for two weeks while on holiday.

The three golden rules I stuck to were: walk at least 10,000 steps a day (or build towards it), eat meals with less than 3 per cent fat whilst keeping an eye on the calories as well. There is a very important thing to remember here and that is keeping one eye on the calorie content and not eating after a curfew in the evening. This is disputed by many but for me having a curfew in an evening means I don't eat, don't consume calories and don't have the problem of not exercising to burn them off. My philosophy with weight loss was that you have to look at three main areas: the head, stomach and feet.

Head: Getting it right and being positive.

Stomach: What you eat.

Feet: Exercise and walking.

I mentioned in the half-time break that breakfast is the most important meal of the day, and it is. Everyone knows it these days. I was straight on to the cereal and semi-skimmed once I started my plan. It's not clever to skip it at all because you are just abusing your body in another way. You've been sleeping for a fair few hours, you've been resting and, once you wake, you need to refuel. It's just like the basic mechanics of running a car, I suppose. Fill it up and it goes, give it the right fuel and it goes on longer, look after it, have it serviced regularly by an expert and it will last a lot longer than just carelessly running it into the ground. But while you can just go out and buy a new car, you can't go out and buy a new you. Once you cash your chips in, that's it. Always eat to refuel via at least three meals a day as well or you'll be running on empty and not performing to the best of your ability.

Don't think you are doing something good and healthy by not eating. It's the wrong way to think. It's crazy talk. Mum always says eat breakfast like a king and supper like a pauper. I'm not sure what you eat like for lunch or dinner ... someone modestly well off but keen not to flaunt it? Just within moderation will see you right. I remember staying at a hotel in Milton Keynes once and they delivered breakfast in a bag and left it outside the room on a morning. I couldn't sleep all night I was getting that excited. Every time I heard a noise I would check outside the room to see if my breakfast had arrived. It was like being tortured. It was a weird system, but that's Milton Keynes for you.

I always lacked structure and that was the first thing I was advised to introduce into my life and my eating. If you don't have structure, you have chaos. You need to have regular meals at regular times, not just an 'I'll eat when I'm hungry or about to pass out' attitude. Food isn't just fuel though. If it was, it would all look and taste the same and we'd have no use for Jamie Oliver. Food should be savoured and enjoyed and chewed properly in comfort. My dad used to say that I ate so fast he could see sparks coming off my knife and folk, and if the truth be known, sometimes I never even tasted the food. How sad is that? What a waste. It's great to see kids enjoying their food. This needs to be encouraged. It's the shovelling in and rushing down of food that needs to be discouraged.

If you have the opportunity to sit down and enjoy a meal with family and friends, make use of it. One reason is that you are given comfort by sitting down at a table; you're not hunched over a plate in front of the TV. It also turns it into a social occasion, which is good for you anyway. I didn't have that many friends and didn't live with my family. I always made time to do this once I realised the benefits, though. And if you cook a meal for friends one night, it leads to them doing the same and keeps it going, maybe even becoming part of your routine. It is also said that overeating occurs less if you eat in company. In this case, make sure to clean everything away so you aren't tempted to pass by the table and pick at food. If you've got kids, there is always the temptation to do the old 'If you don't want it, I'll have it' at mealtimes. I'm not a parent, but it is all about willpower, and I can relate to that. You need discipline ... avoid leftovers by binning them, avoid second helpings by cooking less, avoid big portions by using smaller plates ... there's loads that you can do if you just think a bit about it.

When you are full, leave it. It is better in the waste than on the waist. My problem was always that I didn't know when to stop, it was all about wanting more, needing more – or thinking I did.

Don't just concentrate on food, though. We should be drinking about six to eight glasses (1.2 litres) of water or other fluids every day to stop us getting dehydrated, but avoid drinking soft and fizzy drinks that are high in added sugar. I'm sure we all know that alcohol isn't that good for us by now. There's usually a medical study every few years where a few hundred grand has been spent to tell us that red wine or a glass of stout is good for us in moderation, and the following week, depending on what newspaper you read ... it isn't good for you at all. We know that once we're hammered we get the munchies. Takeaway shops are full on Friday and Saturday nights because of this, not really because everyone actually enjoys kebabs that much. And then the following day it takes forever to get over your hangover, you are dehydrated and have probably eaten everything you can lay your hands on. It certainly is the Demon Drink. You can actually get low-calorie alcohol these days.

For many people, the longest journey starts with the smallest step. My good friend and mentor Dr Chris Steele told me that on the day we first met. I told you he was good with words, didn't I? All of us are guilty of putting something off, saying we'll do it tomorrow. Imagine the productivity, all the things that would get done in the world, the good deeds, the phone calls, the

DIY that would all be resolved if we just did it. I know every excuse about putting something off. I've been there, done it and couldn't even get a T-shirt in my size. At forty-four stone I was probably one of the biggest men in the UK and, yes, I had been on more diets than you can shake a bread stick at.

When you weigh such a large amount it is difficult to comprehend just how much weight you need to lose. You have to take it in small manageable chunks because, let's face it, Rome wasn't built in a day. You know my story, have seen my progress and saw how I went from practically crippled to running the London Marathon in two years.

It is natural for the body to lose weight if you eat less and do more. Every single diet plan in the world is based broadly on this principle. It really is as simple as this. It is important therefore to try and a find a plan that works for you. Plan a diet and create a weight loss plan. That's your next step. Simply saying 'I'm on a diet' doesn't work. You cannot approach it in a half-arsed fashion because you'll have given up within a week. That's all I used to do. I was never really motivated, even when I knew my life was quite at risk. Your plan needs to work for you. My plan worked because it still fitted in with my lifestyle, but I still had to change my lifestyle to fit with the plan as well.

I didn't have structure in my life, so introducing that meant that I was adjusting the way I lived. I ate a healthy breakfast whereas in the past I'd either not had one, or had gone the other way and had a few fry-ups. Planning to have some cereal, with skimmed milk rather than full fat, was making change in moderation. Little changes like changing milks or changing to sweetener rather than sugar if you can't cut it out altogether are small changes that make big differences.

You need to write stuff down. You can only do so much in your head; there's research to be done and figures and menus to prepare. I was always typing details into the computer and coming up with spreadsheets for everything. That's just how my mind works and processes information, but it doesn't mean you have to go into such minute detail. Low-fat foods, creating an eating structure and setting an eating curfew were crucial for me as well. If I was at home and winding down for the night, then I had no way of burning any calories off if I ate a late meal. If you are concerned about anything health-wise in preparation for your plan, ask your doctor about it rather than the 'diet expert' at work (unless you happen to work in a health centre).

Portion control was very important to me; I knew if I was cooking a big meal I would likely eat it in one go. Having a low-fat ready meal sorted this problem out. I didn't get any specialist meals from a health store; these were just the bog-standard healthy choice ready meals you can pick up from any supermarket in the land. They aren't as bad for you as everyone once thought and my weight loss is evidence of this. They were also value for money and I was on quite a limited budget. Just checking the label and seeing it had three per cent in fat or less, it passed my test.

It's important that you get weighed too: what can be measured can be managed. There is no point starting a weight losing plan unless you get weighed first. This is vital. You don't go out to buy something without knowing how much you've got to spend, do you? In the same respect, you can't plan to lose weight when you don't know how much you weigh in the first place! And as you have read, always weigh at the same time, on the same scales, wearing more or less the same clothes.

If you start to obsess and weigh yourself every day it will only lead to disappointment. Remember to tell yourself on day one 'This is the heaviest I will ever be.'

You've read my diet diary. Why not write down your daily thoughts and feelings? Maybe write down what you have eaten, what you have enjoyed and what exercise you have done. I did a spreadsheet on the computer and it was like my own personal weekly magazine of my progress. It really did help and will help you too. Just reading through mine for this book brought back so many memories and feelings – good and bad – but it stands as my journey, showing me where I was, what worked and what didn't. It is just as important to record the elements that don't work for you as the ones that do. Dr Chris said that my plan would have to be changed if the results didn't show and that's why I think it is important to write it all down.

I also think it is important to set goals. I did. I couldn't have done it without them. How do you know what you are aiming for otherwise? Make a wish list; write down everything you want to achieve in life and focus on these things. Make sure they are realistic and achievable. Not all of us can win gold at the Olympics, in fact very few of us can. Make sure your goals are SMART: Specific, Measurable, Achievable, Realistic and Timeable. It sounds like management speak and it is. But it's also weight management speak. To say 'I will lose some weight sometime' isn't a SMART goal whereas 'I will lose five stones within the next six months' is. It sounds dead simple because it is.

At the start of my plan, I couldn't even walk from one side of the living room to the other. There'd have been no way I could have lost so much weight without exercising, though. Most people who rely on diet alone get so far and stall because they're not prepared to get off their backside to burn calories. I understand that everyone has their own circumstances, and I didn't mean that in a bad way, but you really cannot sustain weight loss without moving around a bit.

Get a pedometer and get moving. It's just a small device that fits on to your belt and records the number of steps you make. They are so small that they are easy to lose, sit on and drop down the toilet, so be careful. Write down on a daily basis how many steps you have done (put it in the diary) and don't worry if you don't achieve the magic 10,000 on the first day. When I first started I could hardly make 500. There's no shame in just doing what you can and there's no need to injure yourself. Just keep building it up. I had to walk before I could run too. Vary your walking route if you get bored easily, keep to the streets if you feel vulnerable and get a friend to tag along if you need moral support.

Or join a gym for a couple of grand and go on the walking machine there if you want, as long as you get active. You need to move around to burn calories. If you can jog, then do it, if you want to walk, then walk. You can even get games consoles now to help you get into shape; the key is to introduce some form of exercise into your life that wasn't there before. If you weren't burning the calories before, then a simple walk around the block is a great way to start.

Going out for your first walk can be a bit daunting, especially if you are anywhere near the size I was. So … don't make a big thing of it, just get up and go. But do choose sensible shoes because, believe me, blisters are a nightmare and can easily set you back.

Try to have a small glass of water before you go – but not too much, as you don't want it swilling around or want the loo within five minutes. It's important to

keep hydrated though. It's always best to do some
stretching, even for something as light as walking if
you aren't used to it. Check your watch, know when
you started, and, lastly, open your front door and put
one foot in front of the other ... easy!

Not everyone's boots are made for walking, so here
are a few tips:

Tell someone where (and which way) you are going and
approximately how long you will be.

Walk to a place where you can stop for a break. I walk
to a local supermarket so I can have a quick break and
use the facilities. I call this a pit stop. Going for a walk
isn't just an excuse for walking to the chippy or the pub
though – take it seriously!

Do a reconnaissance mission in advance. Measure
distances and identify landmarks so you are going from
A to B in so many minutes. This is a great way
pacing yourself and measuring improvements. At first
it took me eighty minutes to walk five kilometres, now
I do it in fifty-five minutes, and the improvement gives
me a real sense of achievement.

Warm up and warm down. It's kinder on your body
you start off slow and finish off slow.

If you catch a bus to work (or anywhere), get on the bus
at the next stop along and get off a stop further away.
If you drive, park the car further away. At the shops
park at the far side of the car park. It's a small
difference, but it all counts.

If you think you may get stuck, take your mobile phone

and store a taxi number in it. Or better still, ask a friend to go with you.

Start off with a moderate walk near home and build it up. That way you won't get stranded.

Stick to well-lit, well-used paths.

Book a place on a charity walk or run. It gives you a goal to aim for and there are loads of these organised every year.

Wear appropriate clothing. Living in Manchester, I always have to wear something waterproof.

Exercise was the key for me. There was no way I could have just taken to the streets for a jog even if I'd wanted to. I was determined to walk, though, and there are so many positives surrounding walking that you probably don't even consider unless you are not physically capable of doing it: you don't need to drive anywhere to do it, you can walk at any time you want, is free, you don't need specialist clothing, it's low impact, it is as gentle as you make it, you don't need to announce to the world you are doing it, you can do it with friends for company or use it as alone time or time to catch up on phone calls. You can measure it, you can do it in your lunch hour and you can stop for a break whenever you want. If you have hills nearby, then even better. Build up to it, even go halfway at first. Once you get used to it and if it is safe to do so, have a go at walking up backwards and feel the burn on your legs!

You'd think I enjoy walking the way I go on about it, wouldn't you? At my size, walking was the perfect way to start. Apart from all the benefits to your health, getting out in the open air really makes you feel alive and is good for the soul. Being in the Sunday Club when I was a kid did that for me even though I thought it was worse than torture at the time.

Once you have your plan, your structure and are exercising, stick to it. If you start walking then give it up, you are taking some of that structure away. All of these elements are supposed to work in harmony, so taking one of them away will upset the balance. Importantly, you'll know you are cheating yourself.

Make sure the plan is realistic also. If your eating plan involves six hours of preparation every day is it going to last? If it involves eating foods you don't like, however good they may be for you, will you stick to it? The answer to both questions is probably a big fat no.

Healthy eating, walking and a positive mental attitude are the best way for long-term weight loss. Try to avoid silly faddy diets because they simply don't work. Top celebrities can generally afford personal trainers and surgery. If you can't open a packet of biscuits without eating them all then just don't buy them in the first place.

Nobody else can do this for you – it's all up to you. Everyone is looking for an easy way to lose weight or someone or something to blame for being overweight. Ninety-nine per cent of people who are overweight eat too much and do too little exercise. Some of us are more prone to weight gain than others, and some will find weight loss regimes incredibly difficult (I know I still do). But for most of us, we control our own destiny. Set yourself small weight loss targets and then treat yourself when you achieve them. The treats should be non-food, such as having a holiday, getting your hair done or buying some new clothes. Break the weight you need to lose into small manageable chunks. It doesn't seem that frightening then.

And if you feel like giving up, look at your diary and at old pictures of yourself and see how far you have come. I had help, I had pressure, I made promises, but I'd had all of that before *This Morning* had input. The difference for me was that I didn't do anything the right way until I reached the end of the road and did it to save my life. But you: take it slowly, there's no rush, you'll get there if you stick at it.

Setting personal goals gives you something to aim for and a sense of achievement when you reach them. You need to set ones that are possible otherwise you'll never do it and you'll end up back where you started and feeling like a failure. I made my own list that I could print off and write in:

What I want to achieve	Mission accomplished
Have a bath	yes
Wear socks	yes
Catch a bus	yes
Get on a train	yes
Go to the supermarket	yes
Wear real trousers	yes
Eat out with friends	yes
Walk to work	yes
Do a 10k run	yes
Fly on a plane	yes
Wear a nice suit	yes
Do the London Marathon	yes

By setting realistic goals, I was able to accomplish them all. They are simple, they may be things that everyone takes for granted, but at the time I couldn't do things that everyone took for granted. It worked for me. It also worked for me because I was SMART and had a realistic plan. It has to include a time by which to do it and be something that isn't out of your reach. Make sure that your goals are consistent with others and fit with your immediate and long-range plans too.

When I returned from Australia, I found myself back home and very much at loss as to what I would do with my life. Before I left I'd had a friend, Tamir, staying at my house and, whilst sometimes it was difficult as we suffered with depression, it was great company and stopped me from sitting at home overeating. Overeating has always been a huge danger for me and a very personal thing which I have always done alone. People used to comment that they couldn't understand why I was fat because they'd never seen me eat. This was because I'd do it all in private. I couldn't eat in company and still struggle with it.

Being back at home with the comedown of travelling and the reality of no money, no job and no direction was a dangerous position to be in. This was where I could easily fall off the wagon. Without anyone there I was also back in an isolated environment. It would be like going back to square one if I didn't control it.

I had to think about what I could do in life. I knew that I had a great skill for and enjoyed helping others and I had an unpaid column for the *North West Evening Mail*, but this didn't really offer me the structure I needed. Or the money. I had my own show on Manchester community radio station All FM to provide some structure but this was also an unpaid gig and with the media banging on about the credit crunch every five seconds I needed the kind of gig that would pay my bills.

I was offered a job running my own bingo club in Hyde and, while it was not ideal, it would at least keep the wolf from the door and offer an income. I started on 1 September 2008 and, typically, by then I still hadn't invested in a crystal ball. It was a bad decision that led to me spiralling into depression and falling off the wagon good and proper. Tea breaks were three-hour spectaculars from 3pm until 6pm and I was sometimes left in the club alone with a kitchen crammed with food calling me. It was a very dark time and, despite making some great friends and enjoying some aspects of it all, it was a terrible six-month episode in my life. We do things like this to survive – we take jobs we don't necessarily want and in our minds we tell ourselves *It'll do for now, just till I get back on my feet and get something permanent sorted.*

I was so depressed during this period that I even stopped going out shopping with Beryl. This had been a routine we'd kept to every week for the last couple of years, apart from when I was away. When you start letting the structures in your life just fall by the wayside, you know something is wrong. That's if you can actually see what you're doing. When I was gripped by depression, I could let anyone down and not know. I could be horrible, I could be nasty and I could be very selfish. We all can if we put our minds to it.

Depression gave me a sense of diminished responsibility and extreme paranoia. In December I was invited to a party and, whilst I would normally have jumped at a chance to go to a party, I was fearful that everyone would see that I'd gained weight and this would be too embarrassing for me to endure. I didn't want people looking at me, scrutinising me, commenting on how I'd let myself go, watching what I would eat. I wanted to go to this party feeling like a million dollars and oozing confidence and instead I went to it feeling like I was down and out. I shouldn't have gone. This was the same feeling I used to get in social situations. You know, if I was out with a group of people at a buffet or carvery, I'd always be the one sat there with the smallest portion. I'd feel all eyes on me, I'd know people would be nudging each other, pointing, whispering, without even seeing them doing it. Why? Because, unfortunately, that's what people are like. They'd be watching me to see how much I'd be piling on to my plate and to see how many times I went back for more. I'd hate walking into a room because of the reaction I always got. And it wasn't anything new, remember, I'd had this all my life. In fact, the staring wasn't really that embarrassing anymore, it was boring and tedious. Sometimes I wanted to confront people. 'Yes, I'm fat. Yes, I'm getting some food. Look ... there's my plate. I've just got the same as you, a little bit less, actually,' but what would have been the point?

So, it looks like I was right after all. You may have won the odd battle, but I won the war. If I'm the outright winner, what does that make you? Eh? Come on ... say it!

It makes it even better for me to see all the media coverage you had before piling it all back on. And it's not just the odd pound, it's stones. What now, Mr Healthy Eating expert? Bag of pies and a fish supper washed down with two litres of coke? Look ... there's the phone ... why not order a couple of banquets for two? Pretend you've got friends again for old time's sake, what do you reckon?

You know, Walduck, I was actually scared of you at one point. You were unbeatable. I admired what you were doing. How often can someone say that about

213

you? Once you got going, there was no stopping you. Even when you slipped up a few times, I could tell you were strong. You had determination. No one on the planet had done what you did. You had it all and you threw it away.

It was just a holiday, really. But hey, you got to do a few things that you wouldn't have had a chance to, so at least you got something out of it. You've got your newspaper articles to look back on, you've got the photos of you looking in good nick to bring you back to earth and you've got all those clothes going up in size that you wasted your money on to enjoy on your way back up.

When I was completely under like this, I'd be so scared in the build-up to leaving the house. I never used to go out unless completely necessary. I lost all my confidence. In the past this happened because of the way people used to treat me and sneer. It's like walking past a dog when it knows you are scared of it — it'll sense that fear. I think confidence is quite similar. People pick up on it and take advantage and bully.

I'd try not to go back to my old ways, as you know. It was a daily fight, and I was gripped by depression and barely treading water. One time I just thought that was it and went to the supermarket to get supplies in. Just thinking about it had me excited ... cheese and bread and butter, pies, pasties and cake. I went and bought a couple of bagfuls and when I was on my way home a woman recognised and stopped me.

'You don't know me, but I've seen you on television. You are amazing, and I'm so proud of you,' she said. And as she said it, she leaned in and gently held my face in her hand and stroked my cheek so lovingly. 'You are a wonderful young man.'

Well, that was it. I had a tear in my eye as I walked up the road and felt so bloody guilty that I was carrying all that food. And then again – eating food isn't a crime.

To an extent, it was only after losing weight that I was able to interact sociably. Yes, I spoke to people at work and had workmates, but when I was at work I was on my chair on the stage, behind my calling unit, behind my microphone and I was safe. I was isolated though. I never really spoke to anyone directly and would be there most of the time.

To go back to square one would be a million times worse. I'd have had a taster of what 'normality' was and I'd see it slipping away meal by meal. As an obese man in the past, I knew there was never going to be any chance of me copping off with anyone on a night out. Socialising, drinking, smoking, sex ... the main reasons behind a night out held no interest for me. I was only interested in eating and I wasn't going to go to a bar on a night just to sit and eat crisps or nuts. I couldn't understand the rationale behind it. I wanted to be at home eating, not in a bar.

There was one time I can recall that I did drink. During a period gripped by depression, I wanted desperately to lose weight and felt so alone. I wanted to get out and meet someone. It didn't have to be a life partner; I just wanted to find someone. I have needs too and would have loved to be a bit daring and indulge in a one night stand or two. It doesn't make me a sleaze or anything; it's just a basic need in life that adults have. And lacking in the confidence department, the way forward (so I thought) was to drink alcohol ahead of a night on the town.

I stopped off at the shop on the way for the bus and

bought the cheapest thing I could find ... a bottle of sherry. Being an inexperienced drinker, I just went down a backstreet and necked the whole thing in one and ended up being a lot more confident than I ever imagined. This kind of confidence isn't really that attractive though. I was absolutely hammered. And it only led to wanting to eat when I returned home. I persevered with going out for around four weeks until I gave up. It just wasn't to be. I was just drinking because I couldn't cope with rejection and I thought the alcohol would turn me into Superman.

That's one of the reasons why I've never had a relationship. I certainly would never have the courage to ask anyone out. There's always been low self-esteem in the way too. I've never thought of myself as attractive. I'm sure there's someone out there who thinks so, and would like me, but the biggest hurdle is always yourself. You've got to love yourself before anyone will love you, and all that. It's a big regret to know that I reached the age of forty and had never shared my life with anyone. At all. I'd push people away or get the signals wrong if someone was being kind, thinking they were attracted to me.

In terms of sex I am not saying I am a person who has no sexual experiences at all, but certainly nothing I would want to write about here and certainly nothing of any earth-shattering significance. I'd never been with anyone, never been out on a date with anyone, enjoyed a first kiss, a relationship and certainly never had a one-night stand. Those first weeks and months of meeting someone when life is brilliant, waking up with someone on a morning and feeling secure, commenting on how they look, holding hands in public ... it's a massive list that I thought too great to bother putting on my list of goals that I wanted to achieve. I've

216

struggled with who I am since being an awkward lad and then going through puberty and becoming an awkward teen and then an awkward man. I've wrestled with so many inner demons, feelings and emotions, decisions about who, where and what I am.

I think when I lost weight, I started to see myself for who I am and started to like myself. I definitely started to accept myself and that was one gigantic leap for Walduck kind. I have had a lot of attention from women because of the weight loss. I think this is an attraction not necessarily of how I look, but because of what I've been through. A lot of women have gone through the same thing and can relate to it all. If I'd been that kind of guy, I could have taken advantage of my position like some rock star on tour.

As I write this, it's around three years since I hit my target weight. I still look at myself and there are so many things I don't like. My legs are permanently scarred and will always serve as a reminder of the abuse they endured. I still have wobbly bits that I'll never be happy with. My weight will always be up and down. I've had good spells and bad spells, but I know I'll always keep going. I know I'll always eat instant food if I have it in the house, so I ruled it out of my life. The temptation is always there, always will be.

The last few years have been amazing for me, this goes without saying. I have now completed a journey around the world, lost thirty stones, run four Great North Runs, four Manchester Runs, the London Marathon, climbed the Sydney Harbour Bridge, snorkelled on the Great Barrier Reef, eaten kangaroo in a restaurant in Melbourne, shopped in Singapore, jogged in Central Park and lived my life to the full.

I'm still on All FM, have my own breakfast slot on mancherserradioonline.com, I help out in the bar there too, still get interviewed all the time about health issues and am still a regular guest on *This Morning*. My latest goal is to find employment doing something within the entertainment industry that will pay my way and serve as the ultimate SMART move.

It isn't easy at all to cope with addiction and come through it. Anyone who says it is cannot understand. Life is difficult enough without feeling excluded from society just because of the way you look. I feel I've got the added pressure of scrutiny all the time, like there's an expectation that I'll fall off the wagon and there's so many people waiting to say I told you so. Those people will be around for you too. You cannot let them affect what you are trying to achieve. The smallest and most hate-filled comment can set you back, but why should you let the words of some moron get to you? Remember, there are more good people in the world than the morons.

When I talk at length to people about my food obsession they tell me it is typical addictive behaviour. Being addicted to anything can turn even the most honest person into a deceitful one. Telling lies and deceiving people has never been something I have been comfortable with, but at times I have found myself doing it. For many years, food was in control of me and I still have my moments now when the desire to overeat and hide myself away and binge on food gets the better of me.

I hope by reading this book you will have been inspired that it is possible to turn your life around however bad things get. I hope anyone needing to lose weight will have found some tips and motivation in trying to achieve that goal.

Whatever anyone else might say, reading a book will not make you thin. Nobody can make you thin, other than yourself. I was fortunate that I had some great support around me, but I think that you will find that family and friends will be supportive of you once you show you are serious. In the past I had many attempts at losing weight and, while friends had probably tired of my many attempts, their support was unquestionable once my efforts started to show even the smallest signs of success. That's what friends do – they stick by you and support you.

I will always have a problem with food and I want to be honest about that right here and now. I have always said I may one day end up putting the weight back on, but every time these fears resurface I will read the words I have written in this book, think of the bad times and think in a positive way about the future. I will revisit my wish list and add some new goals. I will keep a check of my food consumption, stick to my golden rules and look at whether I am eating right, cooking right and shopping right. In fact, I am living proof that it works. At one stage in my weight loss programme I got down to thirteen and a half stone, and boy did I look terrible. I took it way too far and looked gaunt, like a bag of bones. I looked ill. I was advised by Dr Chris to put a couple of stones back on. And then when I did, guess what the comments were?

With no other real vices in my life, the only one has always been food, so it stands to reason that I'll go off the rails on occasion. The thing is, now I am aware of it and can control it. I think about food every waking moment. I used to dream about food when I first started losing weight and I still dream about it now. The temptation is always there, so there is always going to be a battle in my life. I'd choose the best meal in the world above the best sex in the world. I'd choose it above anything.

At the back of my mind, I'm always worried that I'll fall off the wagon. Every addict will always feel this, and because I lost the weight in such a public way I'll always feel scrutinised everywhere I go and with every mouthful I eat. There will always be someone looking in my shopping basket, always someone looking at what I eat in a restaurant and always one of them ready to pass comment and judgement.

As I got to the end of the writing this book I had to think long and hard about what words to use to finish it. After all, I want the message to be upbeat. I want you to believe that you could go away and achieve anything you want. I visited Barrow-in-Furness for my Dad's seventieth birthday, and a lot of kids I grew up with were there, including my cousins Russell, Philip, Alistair, Nigel, Robert and Elaine. We had all grown up together and everyone's lives had turned out differently. As I looked around the room, I could see they all now had families of their own and it really made me realise what I had missed out on, not just through my lack of confidence, but mainly because everything was secondary to food ... my addiction, my Achilles heel, my controller. It was great to see all the family and to see my nephews and nieces, friends and family having a great time. It was like looking back to when we were kids, sneaking the odd drink from Mum and Dad, with the world in front of us. At that time, none of us knew what the future was to hold.

I wish I could turn back the clock, but I can't. Nobody can, and as soon as you accept that you can move on. Living differently through hindsight would be easy though – there's always someone you should have said 'I love you' to, a drunken night you regret, forgetting an important date, letting someone down ... we'd all change something if we could. Whatever your age and whatever your circumstances, it is never too late to turn things around. There is always light at the end of the tunnel. Sometimes the tunnel is long and the light is dim, but the journey must start somewhere and it starts with that very important first step.

Thank you for reading the book and good luck in battling your own demons, whatever they might be.

Charles

Acknowledgements

To Dr Chris Steele from *This Morning*, now a personal friend, who helped to give me the strength and motivation to achieve my goal.

To all the production team of *This Morning* (Steve, Justine, Claire, Matt and Steve) who followed me on my journey and who gave me so much endless support.

I would also like to say a special thank you to Fern Britton and Phillip Schofield (the then-presenters of *This Morning*); two wonderful warm people who were especially kind and who helped allay any fears I may have had about appearing on their programme and did all in their power to help me feel comfortable and relaxed.

To all my work colleagues, who shared my ups and downs, frustrations and suffered my mood swings, yet continued to stand by me. Undoubtedly, without their help and co-operation, I would have been unable to continue working.

To my dear friend Lucy, who was so worried about me that she decided to write to *This Morning* and who has always been there for me and still is. Many thanks to my other friends, especially Mark and Beryl.

To Darianne Reay, who helped with the earlier parts of the book. Thanks must also go to the following for providing pictures: Jeremy Durkin, the *Manchester Evening News*, the *North West Evening Mail* and my good pal Gary Taylor.

To Dave Foran, Paul Ripley and radio legend James Stannage for not just giving me the opportunity to present my own breakfast show on Manchester Radio Online but also for giving me some great support and friendship over the last six months. Also thanks to Dannielle Porter and Paul Graham who have given me endless opportunities in radio.

Thanks also to David and Nicola at the Great Run who have been fantastic in getting me involved with the Great Run series and treated me like a real celebrity.

Finally, to everybody who has supported me through e-mails, telephone calls and letters. The depth of feeling and words of encouragement have meant so much to me.

To each and every one of you – my sincere and deepest thanks.

Charles

About the author

Charlie Walduck is a record-breaking slimmer who lives in Failsworth, Manchester. Amongst his jobs, he is most well known for being a bingo caller for several years and now hosts his own radio shows, as well as frequently commenting on obesity issues in the media. He's currently looking for his big break in TV and radio and can be found most days on the URL below.

http://www.facebook.com/charlie.walduck

READ MORE NON-FICTION FROM TONTO BOOKS:

Shakespeare and Love
Raymond Scott with Mike Kelly
Paperback, £7.99, 9780955632693, available April 2010

The Shakespeare First Folio is one of the most revered books in the English language and worth millions. One is owned by billionaire John Paul Getty; another was in the hands of Raymond Scott, who lived with his mum in their modest Tyneside home until his arrest.

When he tried to sell the folio to fund the good life with his young Cuban dancer fiancée, Raymond sparked an international investigation involving the FBI, Interpol and the British police. Did he steal it from Durham University ten years ago, or was he just an innocent middleman for the real owner, a former bodyguard to Fidel Castro?

Shakespeare and Love lifts the lid on this real-life crime mystery, told by the man at the centre of the extraordinary tale – Raymond Scott himself. As he says: 'There are two Raymond Scotts – one who lives quietly at home with his mother, the other who people think is some Raffles-type international thief.'

READ MORE NON-FICTION FROM TONTO BOOKS:

Faces
Bernard O'Mahoney & Brian Anderson
Hardback,   £50.00,   9781907183058,   available
December 2009

Villains, gangsters or 'faces' as they prefer to be called,
are the men, gangs and families that have been
making newspaper headlines for all the wrong reasons
over the past 50 years. Some of their names are
household ones, strangers talk about them as if they
are long lost friends but few people would know them if
their paths crossed in the street. The mere mention of
these people can strike fear into individuals and, in
some cases, communities.

Despite their notoriety, the faces of many of
Britain's most feared criminals remain unknown. That
is until now.

For the very first time, Britain's most infamous
characters and crooks have agreed to be photographed
to appear in a book that will become an important part
of our social history. Forget the so-called 'celebrity
gangster' set that brag and boast about crimes they
dreamt up for inclusion in their memoirs ... forget the
football hooligans that promoted themselves from being
social nuisances into underworld gang bosses ... forget
the steroid enhanced doormen who stuff their bloated
frames into ill-fitting dinner jackets and then tell
anyone who'll listen that they are the Guv'nor.

The people featured in this book are the real deal.
They have been there, done it and have the T-shirt.

READ MORE NON-FICTION FROM TONTO BOOKS:

Sin Cities: Adventures of a Sex Reporter
Ashley Hames
Paperback, £7.99, 9780955632600, available now

With a weakness for women, good times and binge drinking it seemed inevitable that Ashley Hames would turn cult hero with *Sin Cities*, blazing a toxic trail through a minefield of debauchery and fantasy across the globe.

As clown prince of L!VE TV, he happily changed his name by deed poll to News Bunny and produced such lowbrow classics as *Topless Darts*. A few months down the line his career had him hoisted up on meat hooks, tortured, clamped and generally trampled on in the name of entertainment. It was only when the cameras stopped rolling that it got messy.

In this book, Ashley investigates the sexual habits of some of the most extraordinary people on the planet – from the bizarre to the unimaginable – and somehow helps it all make perfect sense.

READ MORE NON-FICTION FROM TONTO BOOKS:

Stephen Miller: Paralympian – My Autobiography
Paperback, £9.99, 9780955632617, available now

Stephen Miller is one of Britain's most successful athletes. Record-breaking Stephen, who has cerebral palsy, is also a writer and poet. Stephen's inspirational autobiography tells of his struggles and triumphs, and is told with refreshing honesty and infectious humour.

'I know how hard it is to compete at the highest level. It takes dedication, courage and self-belief, and Stephen has those qualities in abundance. His story is truly unique and inspiring'

Kevin Keegan, Foreword

The Road to Hell
Sheila Quigley
*Hardback,   £18.99,   9781907183034,   available
November 2009*

DI Lorraine Hunt is back in the next instalment of
Sheila Quig-ley's gritty crime dramas set in Houghton-
le-Spring.

When a woman's body is found mutilated in a field
outside of Houghton-le-Spring, it's more than just
another case for DI Hunt. Not only does the body show
evidence of violation and human bites, it transpires
that Hunt knows the victim. But she also knows that
this is an exact replica of a crime that occurred more
than fifteen years ago, on an evening that changed her
and her friends' lives forever.

With flashbacks to Lorraine's past, The Road to Hell is
a charged, fast-paced page turner with appeal to
Quigley fans old and new.

READ MORE FICTION FROM TONTO BOOKS:

Dirty Leeds
Robert Endeacott
Paperback, £7.99, 9781907183003

1961. Dirty Leeds is a struggling industrialised city in the north of England.

Dirty Leeds is the city's club, sometimes called a football team; its home ground Elland Road, rarely called a stadium.

Dirty Leeds is the label given to Leeds United in 1964 by the FA for improper conduct on the field. Other first teams have far worse disciplinary records, but mud sticks.

Dirty Leeds is where young Jimmy O'Rourke is born and bred, brought up by his grandma in the shadow of the hallowed ground itself. This gives him a thirst for the beautiful game and determination to play for the club he loves.

Dirty Leeds is a hidden history of Don Revie and his men, and the story of Jimmy's dramatic life, from 1961 to 1974.

For information and details on all Tonto Books past,
present and future, please visit the website
www.tontobooks.co.uk